**PUBLISHED**

# FORTHCOMING MONOGRAPHS

**Cardiac Imaging in Adults**
*C. CARL JAFFE, M.D.*

**The Traumatized Hand and Wrist**
*LOUIS A. GILULA, M.D.*

**Imaging Modalities in the Spine**
*MORRIE E. KRICUM, M.D.*

*SAUNDERS MONOGRAPHS in CLINICAL RADIOLOGY*

# Radiology of Orthopedic Procedures, Problems and Complications

VOLUME **24**

MARTIN I. GELMAN, M.D.

Associate Clinical Professor of Radiology
University of Utah
Salt Lake City, Utah

## W. B. SAUNDERS COMPANY

*PHILADELPHIA   LONDON   TORONTO
MEXICO CITY   RIO DE JANEIRO   SYDNEY   TOKYO*

W. B. Saunders Company:    West Washington Square
Philadelphia, PA   19105

1 St. Anne's Road
Eastbourne, East Sussex BN21 3UN, England

1 Goldthorne Avenue
Toronto, Ontario M8Z 5T9, Canada

Apartado 26370—Cedro 512
Mexico 4, D.F., Mexico

Rua Coronel Cabrita, 8
Sao Cristovao Caixa Postal 21176
Rio de Janeiro, Brazil

9 Waltham Street
Artarmon, N.S.W. 2064, Australia

Ichibancho, Central Bldg., 22-1 Ichibancho
Chiyoda-Ku, Tokyo 102, Japan

**Library of Congress Cataloging in Publication Data**

Gelman, Martin I.

Radiology of orthopedic procedures, problems, and complications.

(Saunders monographs in clinical radiology; v. 24)

1. Radiography in orthopedia.    I. Title.    II. Series.
   [DNLM: 1. Bone and bones—Radiography.    W1 SA975B
   v.24 / WE 141 G319r]

RD734.5.R33G44 1984        617'.3        84–5345

ISBN 0–7216–4079–6

Radiology of Orthopedic Procedures, Problems and Complications    ISBN   0–7216–4079–6

Last digit is the print number:    9    8    7    6    5    4    3    2

To my parents, Ray and Samuel, who toiled to give me the opportunity.

To my loving wife, Sheila, and my children, Lisa, Stephanie, and Andrew, for whose patience, support, and reassurance I am eternally grateful, and whom I can never repay.

# PREFACE

The impetus to write this text arose from a need recognized while teaching orthopedic radiology over a 10-year period to residents in radiology, physical medicine and rehabilitation, rheumatology, and orthopedic surgery. The focus of this work, therefore, is to provide, in a single, easily used source, practical information and explanations regarding the more common orthopedic problems confronted by the radiologist and orthopedic surgeon. More current ancillary radiologic modalities such as radionuclide scanning, computed tomography, and arthrography have been included in those areas where they contribute significantly to problem solving or patient management.

This text is intended to be kept in the radiology reading room and to be utilized as a ready reference, but by no means is it meant to be exhaustive. As with any significant undertaking, a long-term commitment should be fulfilled. It is sincerely hoped that this volume will provide and enable greater communication and understanding between the radiologist and orthopedic surgeon, so that through meaningful dialogue the radiologist will understand what is important to the orthopedic surgeon and the orthopedic surgeon will avail himself of the talents and procedures the radiologist has to offer.

MARTIN I. GELMAN, M.D.

# ACKNOWLEDGMENTS

I would like to acknowledge my teachers in the field of radiology who made this book a reality. My sincere thanks to Dr. Philip J. Hodes and Dr. Jack Edeiken, who gave me the tools with which to work. I am indebted to my colleagues in skeletal radiology, orthopedic surgery, and rheumatology, too numerous to mention individually, for their academic support, teaching, and friendship.

A number of individuals have worked in collaboration with me in the preparation of this book. Mr. Julian Maack, Director of Medical Illustration at the University of Utah Medical Center, is responsible for the medical art work, and his staff for the medical photography and photographic prints. I would like to thank Ms. Patricia Mavor, Mrs. Constance Staples Ward, Mrs. Rebecca Harris, and Mrs. Evalyn Christensen for their help, cooperation, and expertise in typing the manuscript as the book evolved. Finally, a very special thanks to Ms. Lisette Bralow, Associate Medical Editor at W. B. Saunders Company, for her patience, support, expert guidance, and valued friendship.

# CONTENTS

# 1

# FRACTURES AND FRACTURE HEALING

Radiographic evaluation of a fracture may utilize many descriptive terms. It should, however, convey an accurate assessment of the injury to the orthopedic surgeon. The following parameters, if present, should be commented upon in order to create a "word picture" that communicates the mechanical alteration that has occurred (Table 1–1).

## FRACTURE TERMINOLOGY

*Displacement* refers to the loss of anatomic alignment of fracture fragments in a medial-lateral or anterior-posterior direction. It is described in reference to the distal fracture fragment.

*Distraction* is the separation of fracture fragments. In general, bone heals best in apposition, so distraction is undesirable.

*Angulation* is the degree of angular deformity measured at the fracture site; it is described in reference to the direction that the apex of the angle is pointing (anterior or posterior, medial or lateral). Angulation is

**Table 1–1.** TERMINOLOGY USED IN RADIOGRAPHIC DESCRIPTION OF FRACTURES

Displacement
Distraction
Angulation
Comminution
Transverse or Oblique
Over-riding
Closed or Open
Rotation

more significant in adults than in children because of decreased ability to remodel. The amount of angulation acceptable depends upon whether the plane of angulation corresponds to the plane of greatest motion at the nearest joint and if it is in a weight-bearing bone. As an example, anteroposterior angulation in the lower tibia is better tolerated than medial-lateral angulation because this is the plane of greatest motion in the ankle, which can subsequently compensate for it (Fig. 1–1). Anterior angulation of 15 degrees in the femoral shaft is acceptable, as it can be well compensated for by knee and hip motion. Similar lateral angulation is unacceptable because of the excessive stress forces it will later place on the knee. Lack of compensation by the nearest joint may result in the development of early degenerative arthritis by that joint. Angulation may be corrected by wedging of the cast (Fig. 1–2). Greater angulation is acceptable in the child because of the extensive remodeling that occurs.

*Comminuted* refers to the existence of two or more fracture fragments.

*Transverse* or *oblique (spiral)* refers to a horizontal or oblique fracture line, respectively. In general, oblique or spiral fractures result from indirect force applied to the bone and exhibit less displacement than transverse fractures, which are largely the result of a direct force and are more frequently associated with significant displacement. The more significant factors affecting fracture healing include initial displacement of the fracture, comminution, soft tissue dam-

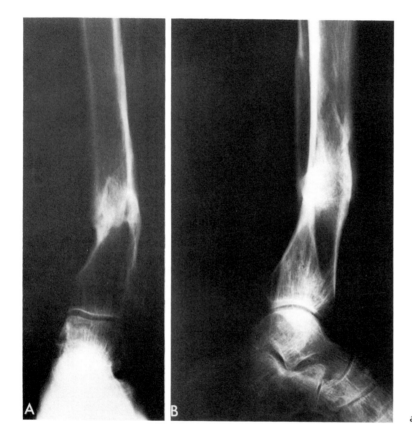

**Figure 1–1.** Anterior and lateral angulation of the distal tibia.

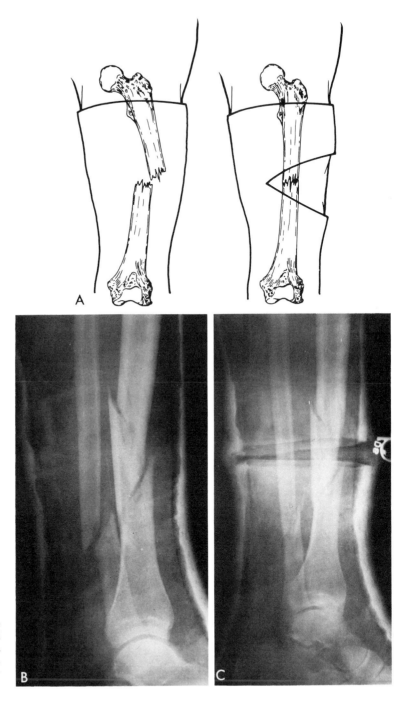

**Figure 1–2.** Wedging of the cast may correct an angulated deformity at the fracture site. *A*, Diagram. *B*, Posterior angulation. *C*, Angulation corrected by wedging of cast.

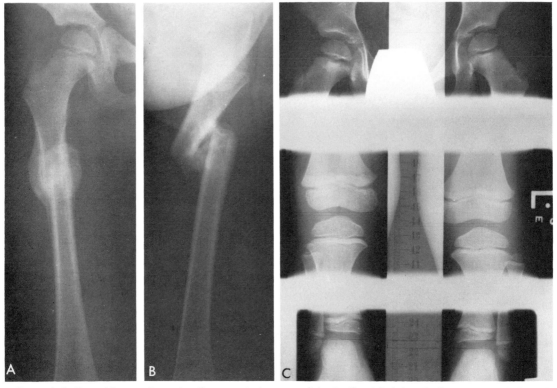

**Figure 1–3.** Over-riding or shortening if uncorrected may result in significant limb-length discrepancy as indicated by scanogram.

age, and interval development of infection.[1, 2, 3]

*Over-riding* (shortening) is the amount of overlap of fracture fragments. This is important because of the resultant shortening of the extremity that may occur if not corrected (Fig. 1–3).

*Closed* (simple) or *open* (compound) describes intact or disrupted skin at the fracture site.

*Rotation* is the displacement of a fracture fragment around a vertical axis (Fig. 1–4).

## HEALING

Radiographically, healing may be assessed by the demonstration of callus and/or gradual obliteration of the fracture line in bones where callus formation is minimal. Although in the acute stage of a fracture the margins are sharp, these become indistinct by approximately the twentieth day owing to hypervascularity and resorption of bone.

It is important to note, however, that the radiographic changes may lag behind the actual clinical situation and that the orthopedic surgeon may allow weight bearing on the clinical basis of no pain over the fracture site, even though the fracture does not appear radiographically to be completely healed.

Callus formation consists of bridging (internal) callus and buttressing (external) callus (Fig. 1–5). When metallic fixation is utilized, healing is most dependent on bridging callus because there is little or no buttressing callus formation (Fig. 1–6). Therefore, if significant periosteal reaction or buttressing callus is observed at the site of a fracture fixed internally, this may indicate motion or infection (Fig. 1–7). A bone graft at the fracture site, however, will promote bridging and buttressing callus formation (Fig. 1–8). Radionuclide scanning, although experimental at present, may provide a means in the future for evaluating fracture healing.[4, 5]

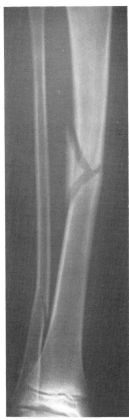

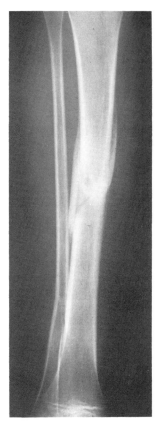

**Figure 1–4.** Rotation of fracture fragments, although significant, is at times difficult to assess. Rotated "butterfly fragment" demonstrates thicker cortex than adjacent bone.

**Figure 1–5.** Bridging and buttressing callus formations are usually observed following closed reduction of a fracture.

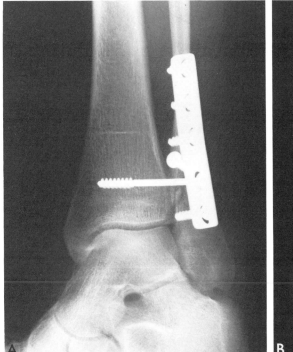

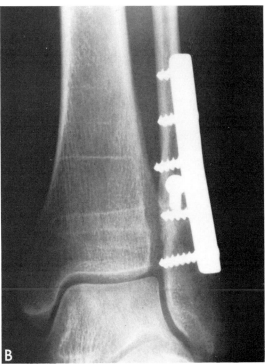

**Figure 1–6.** Bridging callus is primarily responsible for fracture healing when metallic fixation is utilized.

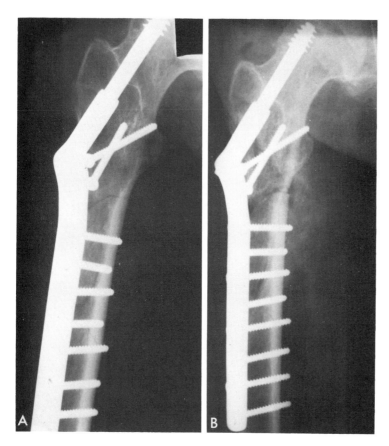

**Figure 1–7.** The presence of buttressing callus or periosteal reaction when internal fixation has been utilized may indicate motion or infection at the fracture site. *A,* Internal fixation of an intertrochanteric and subtrochanteric fracture. *B,* Air in soft tissues, widening of fracture line, and excessive soft tissue callus should suggest infection (*Enterobacter* was cultured).

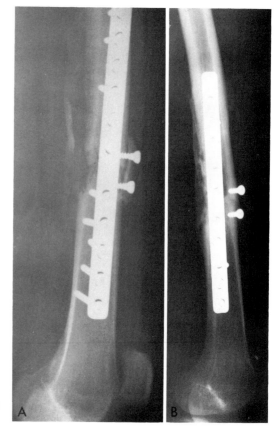

**Figure 1–8.** Bone grafting of a fracture will promote bridging and buttressing callus formation.

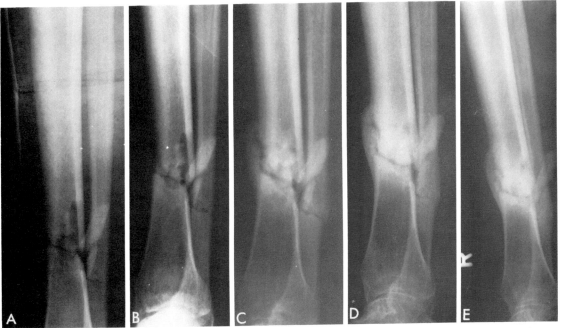

**Figure 1–9.** Delayed union, commonly a clinical diagnosis, is indicated radiographically by a slower-than-usual rate of healing. This sequence occurred over an interval of one and one half years.

## DELAYED UNION VERSUS NONUNION

*Delayed union* is a temporal situation in which healing is occurring in a physiologic manner but at a slower pace than usual. Interval radiographs may show little if any progressive healing; however, delayed union is most commonly a clinical diagnosis substantiated by persistent pain at the fracture site (Fig. 1–9). *Nonunion* is a pathologic state indicated by complete failure of fracture healing. It is characterized radiographically by rounding, sclerosis, and flaring of the bone ends (Fig. 1–10). Delayed union or nonunion may be caused by distraction, extensive surgical dissection, infection, decreased or loss of blood supply, metabolic factors, and inadequate immobilization. The incidence of nonunion in the long bones varies from the highest to the lowest as follows: tibia, radius, femur, humerus, ulna, and clavicle.

## BONE GRAFT

The bone graft may be utilized prophylactically or curatively to promote healing of

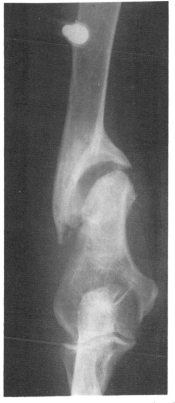

**Figure 1–10.** Nonunion is characterized radiographically by widening of the fracture line, rounding or mushrooming of the fracture margins, and sclerosis.

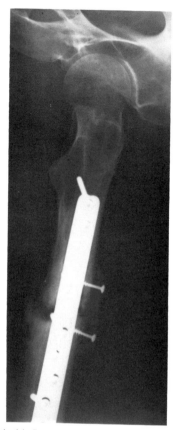

**Figure 1–11.** Bone grafts to promote fracture healing are frequently screwed in place to insure fixation. Note two anterior cortical bone graft screws.

a fracture which undergoes delayed union or nonunion and is frequently fixed in place by metallic screws (Fig. 1–11). It stimulates osteoblastic activity but undergoes necrosis itself and is eventually replaced by new bone. Bone grafts may also be utilized in promoting spinal fusions as well as providing replacement of long bones following such procedures as surgical excision of a tumor (e.g., distal radius replaced by proximal fibula) (Fig. 1–12). Bone grafts or transplants may be classified as any of the following:

*Autograft.* A graft taken from one site and implanted in another in the same individual (e.g., musculopedicle bone graft taken from quadratus femoris muscle along with the bone and blood supply under it to promote femoral neck fracture healing).

*Homograft* (allograft). A graft transplanted from one individual to another of the same species but with different genetic patterns.

*Heterograft* (xenograft). A graft transplanted from an individual of one species to an individual of another species.

## RADIOGRAPHIC ASSESSMENT OF FRACTURES AND FRACTURE HEALING

The goal of fracture treatment is to establish bony union with anatomic position of fracture fragments and restoration of normal function. The radiographic report should be objective in anatomic description without judgmental statements. Remodeling and growth in children may compensate for errors in alignment and even to some degree for shortening, allowing the orthopedist to accept a less than optimal reduction. Radiographs made through a plaster cast may be assessed for alignment; however, they are not adequate for evaluation of the degree of callus formation, and if this is desired, the cast should be removed. Anteroposterior and lateral views are usually sufficient to demonstrate alignment as well as healing; additional views such as oblique or tangential views, however, may be required for adequate evaluation.

Follow-up fracture films should be technically comparable in projection and centering. This is extremely important when evaluating for rotation of fracture fragments, since an oblique projection may falsely suggest rotation of the fragments. This may be obviated by including both ends of the bone on the film and determining whether the rotation is due to patient positioning or the bony fragments themselves (Fig. 1–13). Noncomparable positioning or projections will also erroneously make alignment appear to change from film to film.

In addition to evaluating alignment of bony fragments and healing, careful observation of fixation devices should be made with respect to bony engagement, change in position or bending, fatigue fractures of metallic plates, screws, or devices, migration of fixation devices, and bone resorption indicating loosening secondary to motion of the device or infection (Figs. 1–14 to 1–20) (Table 1–2). Metallic fixation devices and

*Text continued on page 15*

**Table 1–2.** RADIOGRAPHIC FEATURES OF COMPLICATIONS OF ORTHOPEDIC FIXATION DEVICES

Lack of bony engagement of device
Change in position or bending of device
Fatigue fractures of metallic plate, screw, or device
Migration of fixation device
Bone resorption around device indicating loosening secondary to motion or infection

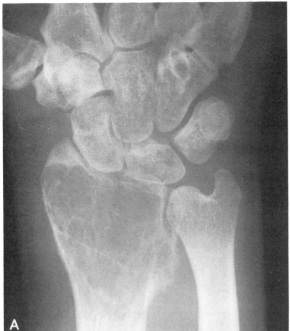

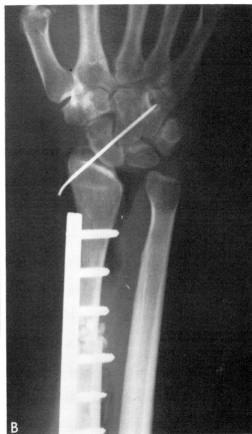

**Figure 1–12.** This giant cell tumor of the distal radius was treated by resection of the distal radius and interposition and grafting of the proximal fibula.

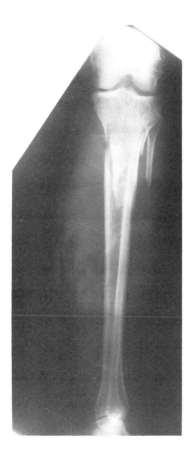

**Figure 1–13.** Inclusion of the knee and ankle joints on the radiograph indicates a well-positioned radiograph with obvious rotation of the lower leg and foot.

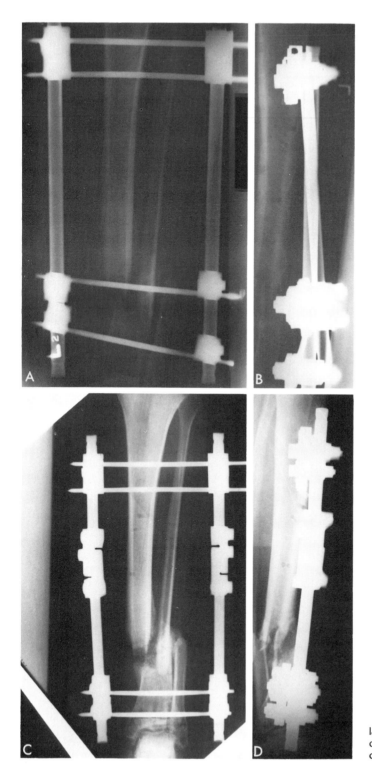

**Figure 1–14.** Initial views demonstrated lack of inferior tibial pins passing through distal tibia. Subsequent films demonstrate correction.

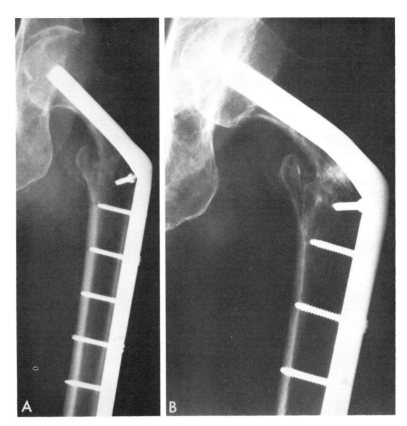

**Figure 1–15.** Bending of this nail with associated increased varus deformity at the fracture site indicates excessive loading at the fracture site.

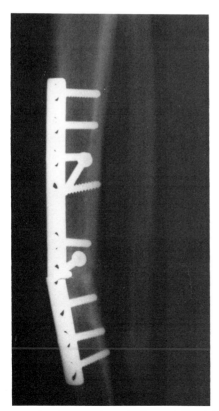

**Figure 1–16.** Fracture through the metallic plate occurred as a result of malpositioning of the plate. The solid portion of the plate should be adjacent to the fracture.

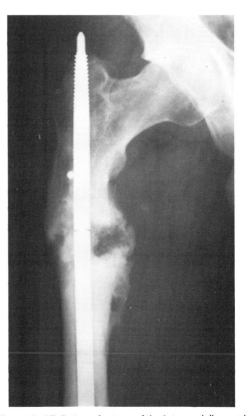

**Figure 1–17.** Fatigue fracture of the intramedullary rod.

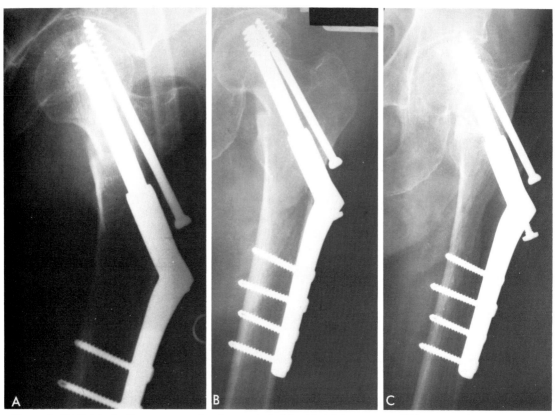

**Figure 1–18.** Originally, the more superior pin penetrated the hip joint at surgery *(A)* but was subsequently pulled back *(B)*. As usually occurs, the pin remigrated into the joint and eroded the acetabular side of the joint *(C)*.

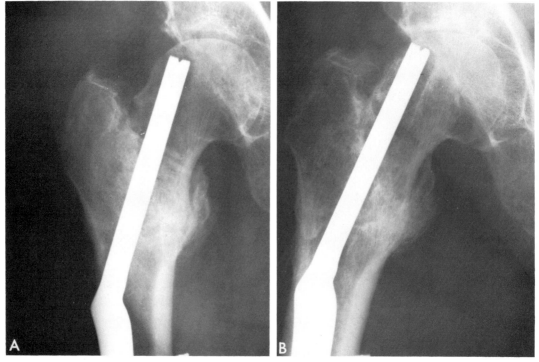

**Figure 1–19.** Resorption of bone around the fixation device over an interval in this patient was due to infection.

12

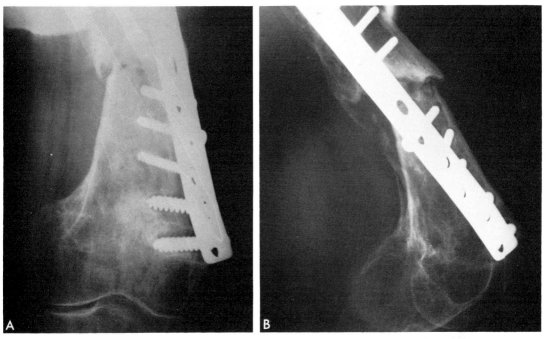

**Figure 1–20.** Resorption of bone around the screws was due to motion and instability.

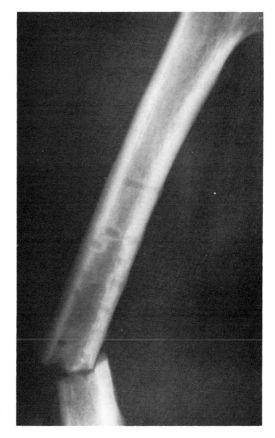

**Figure 1–21.** A fracture may occur through a previous pin or screw hole that has not had time to heal.

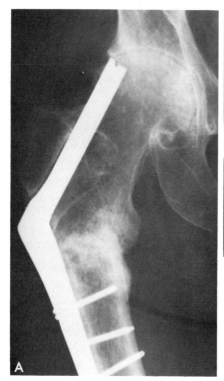

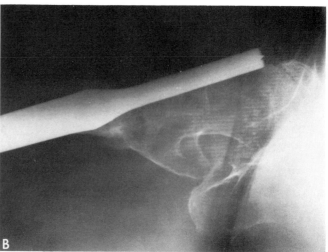

**Figure 1–22.** Jewett nail is noted anterior to femoral head and neck on lateral view.

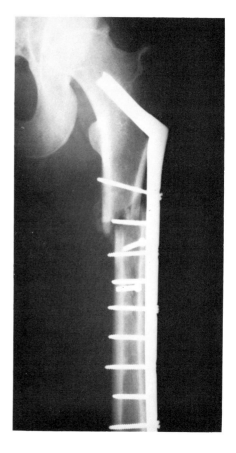

**Figure 1–23.** Screw threads at the fracture site may cause distraction of the fracture fragments.

screws are not usually removed in older patients unless they cause pain, whereas they are usually removed in the younger active patient because they serve as stress concentrators and may cause the adjacent bone to fracture. Previous pin or screw holes, prior to healing, may also allow the bone to fracture (Fig. 1–21). If an orthopedic device is observed beyond bony confines on only one radiographic view, it should still be considered outside of the bone (Fig. 1–22). In screw fixation of fractures, the threads of the screw should be beyond the fracture site in order to allow compression of fracture fragments. If the threads are at the fracture site, they may cause distraction of the fragments (Fig. 1–23). Bending of a nail indi-

cates overloading at the fracture site before it can tolerate such stresses.

## References

1. Nicoll EA: Fracture of the tibial shaft. A survey of 705 cases. J Bone Joint Surg 46B:373–387, 1964
2. Ellis H: Disabilities after tibial shaft fractures. J Bone Joint Surg 40B:190–197, 1958
3. Weissman SL, Herold HZ, Engelberg M: Fractures of the middle two-thirds of the tibial shaft. Results of treatment without internal fixation in 140 consecutive cases. J Bone Joint Surg 48A:257–267, 1966
4. Gumerman LW, Fogel SR, Goodman MA, Hanley EN Jr, Kappankakas GS, Rutkowski R, Levine G: Experimental fracture healing: Evaluation using radionuclide bone imaging. Concise communication. J Nucl Med 19:1320–1323, 1978
5. Wahner HW: Radionuclides in the diagnosis of fracture healing. J Nucl Med 19:1356–1358, 1978

# 2

# THE THORACOLUMBAR SPINE

## TRAUMA TO THE THORACOLUMBAR SPINE

Most fractures of the thoracolumbar spine are not associated with neurologic deficit; however, proper management and treatment depend upon demonstration of the extent of bony and soft tissue injury to prevent subsequent or progressive neurologic deficit. The lumbar spine is highly susceptible to fracture or dislocation because it is located between relatively more stable regions of the spine, i.e., the thoracic and sacral spine. This is reflected in the fact that more than 50 per cent of all vertebral body fractures occur from T-12 to L-2 and about 40 per cent of all spinal cord injuries are at the T-12 to L-1 level.

### Anatomy

An understanding of the anatomy of the spine will allow greater appreciation of the biomechanical response of the spine to trauma. The thoracolumbar spine is a curved column, which is lordotic in the lumbar region and kyphotic in the thoracic region. The vertebral bodies become progressively larger in a craniad-caudad direction and each disc becomes larger and thicker except for the lumbosacral disc, which is usually thinner. Each disc, consisting of a central gelatinous nucleus pulposus and peripheral fibrocartilaginous annulus fibrosus, functions as a shock absorber. In addition to the intervertebral disc, the vertebral end plates may dissipate stress applied to the spine by forcing blood out of the cancellous bone

through multiple vascular foramina. The vertebral end plate will always fail before rupture of the annulus in the normal spine.

The *thoracic spine* (Fig. 2–1) is distinguished anatomically by the presence of ribs. The *head of each rib* articulates on either side of the intervertebral disc with two small facets, one on each vertebral body. The *tubercle of the rib* articulates with the anterior tip of the transverse process of the vertebra. The configuration of the thoracic cage as

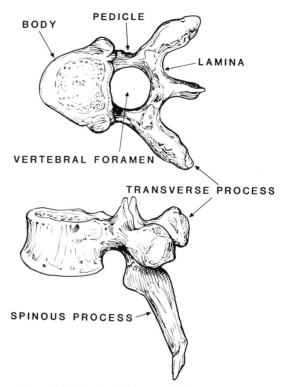

**Figure 2–1.** Anatomic features of the thoracic spine.

16

well as associated articulations restricts lateral bending, flexion, and extension but allows torsion. In addition, the wide laminae in association with the shortened interlaminar ligaments further contribute to the immobility of the thoracic spine.

The lumbar spine is distinguished anatomically by the massive vertebral bodies and posterior processes (Fig. 2–2). The thicker intervertebral discs allow greater mobility as do the longer interlaminar, interspinous, and supraspinous ligaments.

Structurally, the spine may be divided into anterior and posterior columns, which becomes important when determining the potential of an injury in producing acute instability. The anterior column consists of the vertebral bodies, discs, and ligaments, while the posterior column includes the neural arches, facet joints, and ligaments. The *posterior ligament complex* consists of the supraspinal and interspinal ligaments, the facet joints and the ligamentum flavum.[2] The anterior and posterior longitudinal ligaments join the anterior and posterior surfaces of the vertebral bodies, respectively. The interspinal ligament connects the spinous processes and unites posteriorly with the supraspinal ligament, which joins the tips of the spinous processes. The ligamentum flavum contributes toward spinal stability by joining adjacent laminae (Fig. 2–3).[3] Acute instability occurs if both structural columns are disrupted.

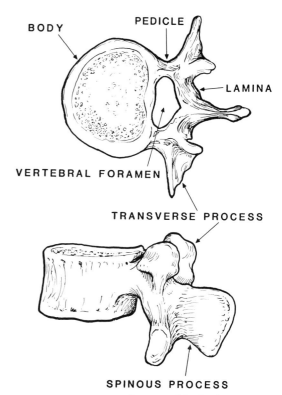

**Figure 2–2.** Anatomic features of the lumbar spine.

## Spinal Stability

**Acutely Unstable Spine.** The acutely unstable spine is capable of motion at the level of injury with subsequent neurologic im-

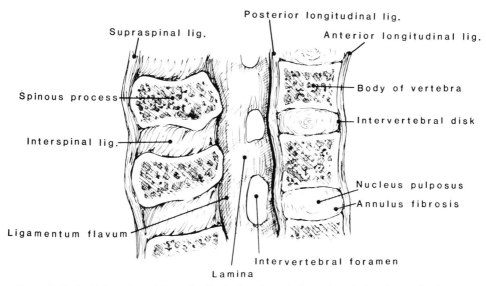

**Figure 2–3.** Sagittal section of the spine illustrating the anterior and posterior structural columns.

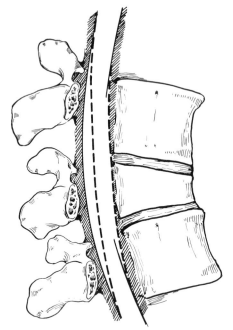

**Figure 2–4.** Increasing kyphosis in the chronically unstable spine may cause compression of the spinal cord.

pairment shortly after injury. All thoracolumbar dislocations and fracture dislocations therefore render the spine acutely unstable. Although both linear and angular displacements may cause neurologic damage, linear displacement is more serious since it may compromise the spinal canal to a greater degree.

**Chronically Unstable Spine.** The chronically unstable spine is capable of slowly progressive increasing angular deformity over a period of months or years. Neurologic sequelae are not common but may occur when the angular deformity is marked (Fig. 2–4).

### Biomechanics of Spinal Trauma

Thoracolumbar fractures or dislocations most commonly result from indirect trauma applied to the spine, causing it to bend in a direction it does not normally go. The force applied to the spine as a result of trauma may be *angular* or *linear*. The *angular forces* include *flexion* and *extension*, *lateral bending*, and *rotation* (Fig. 2–5A). *Nonangular* or *linear forces* include *shear* in an anterior, posterior, or lateral direction, *compression*, and *distraction* (Fig. 2–5B).[1, 2]

*Flexion* injuries, the most common injuries involving the thoracic and lumbar spine, are rarely associated with neurologic damage and are stable. Since the axis of flexion is normally about the center of the intervertebral disc, and since the distance from this axis to the posterior column is three to four times that from the axis to the anterior vertebral body, the force applied to the anterior vertebral body is three to four times that applied to the posterior elements or ligaments, resulting in a wedge-shaped fracture (Fig. 2–6).

*Hyperextension*, although an extremely common cause of fracture and dislocation in the cervical spine, is a very rare cause of injury in the thoracolumbar spine.

*Lateral bending* may produce a lateral wedge fracture, which is similar to the anterior wedge fracture produced by hyperflexion. This fracture is uncommon, most often occurs in the midlumbar region, is stable, and is not usually associated with neurologic deficit.

The thoracolumbar junction represents a transitional area with respect to anatomy and stress. The normal spinal curvature curves from kyphosis into lordosis at this level, permitting increased stress concentration. In addition, the anatomic differences between the thoracic and lumbar vertebrae permit greater rotational mobility, allowing fractures in which rotation plays a role. *Rotation* rarely causes a fracture by itself but combines with flexion as the most common cause of dislocation or fracture-dislocation in the thoracolumbar spine.[4] An oblique fracture of the vertebral body with lateral displacement on the anteroposterior view is evidence of rotation, whereas anterior wedging of the vertebral body on the lateral view indicates the influence of flexion (Fig. 2–7). A variant of this type of injury has been termed the *slice fracture dislocation* by Holdsworth[5] and is predominantly a rotation type of injury and very unstable.

*Shear* force in an anterior, posterior, or lateral direction produces a highly unstable injury that is frequently associated with neurologic deficit. The dislocation of the spine seen in Figure 2–8 cannot be explained by flexion-rotation, since there is no evidence of rotational displacement or of a wedge fracture of the vertebral body but rather by anteroposterior shear. The *shear injury* and *flexion rotation injury* are the most unstable

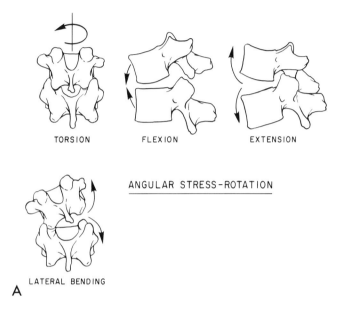

TORSION          FLEXION          EXTENSION

ANGULAR STRESS-ROTATION

LATERAL BENDING

A

**Figure 2–5.** *A*, Angular forces applied to the spine. *B*, Linear forces applied to the spine.

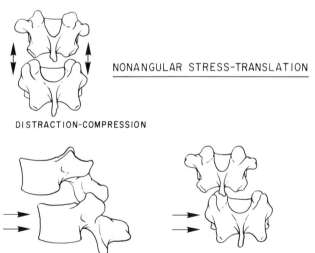

NONANGULAR STRESS-TRANSLATION

DISTRACTION-COMPRESSION

ANTEROPOSTERIOR SHEAR        LATERAL SHEAR

B

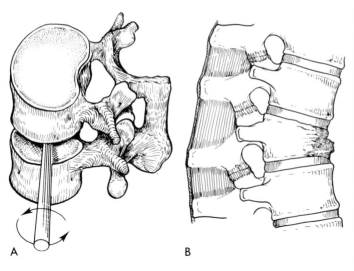

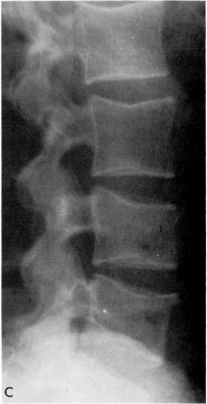

**Figure 2–6.** *A,* Flexion fractures of the spine result from excessive force applied to the anterior vertebral body because the axis in flexion is normally in the center of the intervertebral disc. *B* and *C,* Diagram and radiograph of flexion fractures. (*A,* From Gelman MI, Umber JS: Fractures of the thoracolumbar spine in ankylosing spondylitis. AJR *130*:485–491, 1978.)

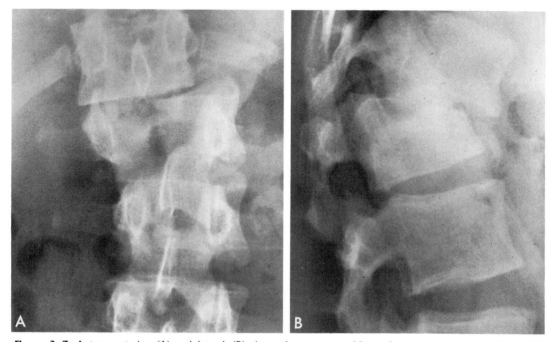

**Figure 2–7.** Anteroposterior *(A)* and lateral *(B)* views demonstrate oblique fracture line, lateral and posterior displacement of the vertebral body, and anterior wedging indicating rotation and flexion forces.

vertical fracture line as the vertebral body is split apart by the invading disc material. In these cases, the posterior portion of the vertebral body may be displaced into the spinal canal, producing neurologic deficit.[5]

*Distraction fractures* are not common but are usually seen in patients who are wearing a lap type of seat belt at the time of injury. Normally the axis of flexion and extension of the spine is somewhere near the center of the intervertebral disc, as mentioned in the discussion of flexion injuries. In seat belt injuries, the axis of flexion is shifted anteriorly to the point of contact between the seat belt and the anterior abdominal wall. The entire spine, being posterior to this axis, is subjected to tensile (distraction) force as the body flexes over the seat belt. The posterior elements of the spine, being furthest from the axis of flexion, typically are distracted a greater amount than the more anterior vertebral body (Fig. 2–10). The dis-

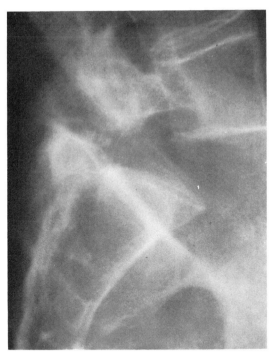

**Figure 2–8.** An anteroposterior shear force resulted in linear displacement of L-5 on S-1. (From Gelman MI, Umber JS: Fractures of the thoracolumbar spine in ankylosing spondylitis. AJR *130*:485–491, 1978.)

injuries incurred by the spine, and neurologic damage is common.

*Compression fractures* (Fig. 2–9) resulting from excessive vertical load are most common in the midlumbar region and are stable. When the compressive force is extreme, the depressed end plates may be united by a

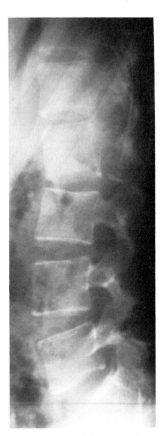

**Figure 2–10.** Widening of the posterior aspect of the L-2 to L-3 disc space indicates a distraction fracture secondary to hyperflexion of the spine. Note also the asymmetry of the corresponding neural foramen and an avulsion fracture fragment.

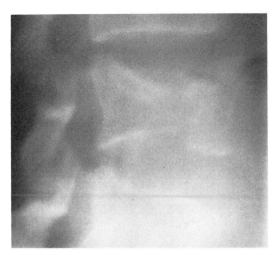

**Figure 2–9.** Lateral tomogram demonstrates vertical fracture through the end plates and vertebral body indicating a compressive force.

traction or tensile force may result in disruption of spinal continuity through bone, soft tissue support, or a combination of both. The pure distraction fracture through bone (Chance fracture) appears the more stable variety, whereas the ligamentous fracture is more unstable.[6, 7, 8, 9] Similarly, fractures have been observed in patients with long-standing ankylosing spondylitis, either through the disc space or vertebral body with extension into the posterior elements (Fig. 2–11). The biomechanics are somewhat similar to those of the seat belt injury in that the ankylosing process effectively shifts the axis of flexion of the spine

anterior and the axis of extension posterior to its normal location in the center of the nucleus pulposus (Fig. 2–12). Radiographic recognition in such patients presenting with sudden focal pain and tenderness is important for selection of proper therapy. External support by a brace may eliminate pain and promote bony healing; if irregularity and sclerosis begin to develop, however, a pseudarthrosis rather than a pyogenic or granulomatous infection should be suspected (Fig. 2–13). This is especially true in the presence of an associated posterior element fracture. Rigid internal fixation and surgical fusion may then be indicated (Fig. 2–14). Although

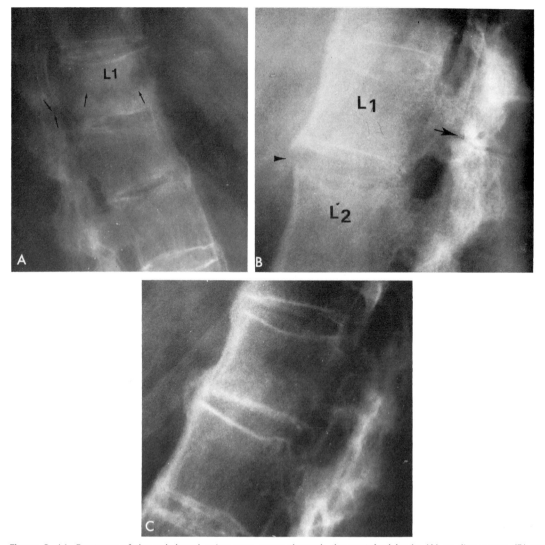

**Figure 2–11.** Fractures of the ankylosed spine may occur through the vertebral body *(A)* or disc space *(B)* and extend through the fused posterior elements (arrows). *C,* Healing may occur spontaneously. (*B* and *C,* From Gelman MI, Umber JS: Fractures of the thoracolumbar spine in ankylosing spondylitis. AJR *130*:485–491, 1978.)

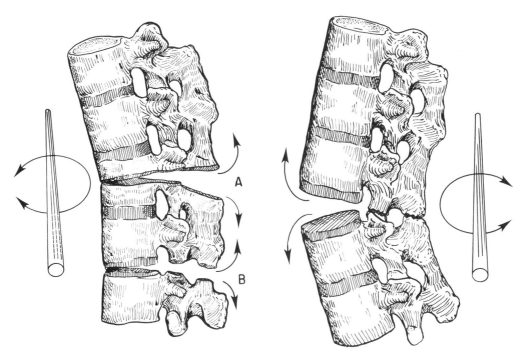

**Figure 2–12.** Ankylosis of the anterior and posterior structural columns of the spine shifts the axis of flexion and extension anteriorly and posteriorly, respectively, from its normal location in the center of the nucleus pulposus. (From Gelman MI, Umber JS: Fractures of the thoracolumbar spine in ankylosing spondylitis. AJR *130*:485–491, 1978.)

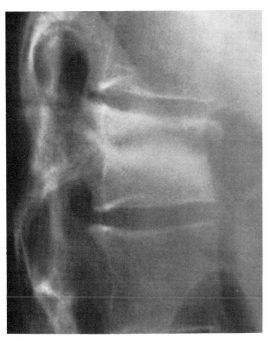

**Figure 2–13.** Irregularity and sclerosis at the fracture site may simulate infection; however, extension of the fracture through the posterior elements clarifies the diagnosis.

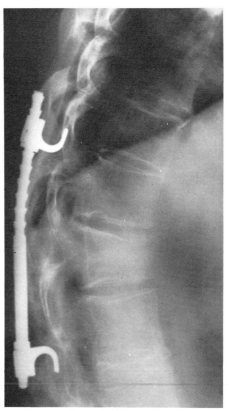

**Figure 2–14.** Although healing may occur spontaneously, rod fixation and surgical fusion may be required (same patient as in Fig. 2–15). (From Gelman MI, Umber JS: Fractures of the thoracolumbar spine in ankylosing spondylitis. AJR *130*:485–491, 1978.)

these fractures have the potential to become unstable, neurologic deficit is usually not present and spontaneous healing may occur.[10]

*Transverse process fractures* are frequently multiple, result from violent muscle pull, and should alert the physician to the possibility of retroperitoneal hemorrhage.[11]

## Radiographic Evaluation

Radiographic evaluation is performed to determine the extent of injury; more specifically, is there encroachment on the spinal cord and canal, at what level, and does the injury make the spine potentially unstable, i.e., are both the anterior and posterior structural columns involved? A vertebral fracture may be quite stable, however, and still cause significant neurologic damage owing to bony impingement of the cord. In addition, a patient who has sustained trauma to the spine may have more than one fracture that is not contiguous, and therefore total spine radiography is recommended as part of the evaluation.[12, 13] An extremely important concept to keep in mind is that the more unstable the spine following an injury, the more unlikely that this may be recognized radiographically because of spontaneous reduction while the patient is in the supine position.[14] It is the function of the radiologist, therefore, to recognize and report the *potential* for acute instability or motion by analyzing the extent of damage to the anterior and posterior columns of the spine.

*Anteroposterior* and *cross-table lateral views* constitute the minimum examination and, although some individuals advocate obliques by careful positioning of film and tube without moving the patient, *hypocycloidal polytomography* appears to be more useful, especially in assessing the posterior column. Thin polytomographic sections have been particularly helpful in demonstrating the entire extent of the fracture (Fig. 2–15). Although tomography may be performed in both the anteroposterior and lateral projections, the lateral projection is essential not only to delineate anterior and posterior column injury but also to demonstrate the extent of compression of the spinal canal (Fig. 2–16).[13] Specifically, the radiographic changes to be sought include *comminution, displacement of the posterior cor-*

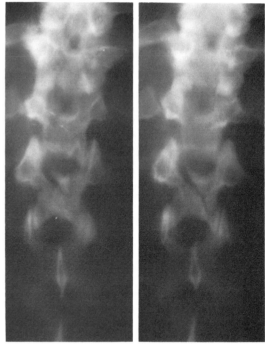

**Figure 2–15.** Successive polytome cuts, 3 mm apart, demonstrate the extent of fracture through the lamina and neural arch.

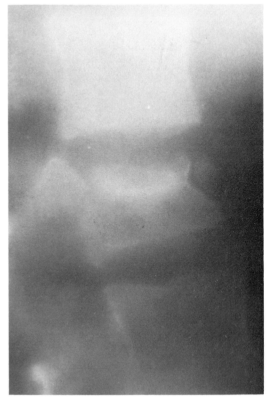

**Figure 2–16.** Tomography in the lateral projection is essential to demonstrate the extent of encroachment on the spinal canal.

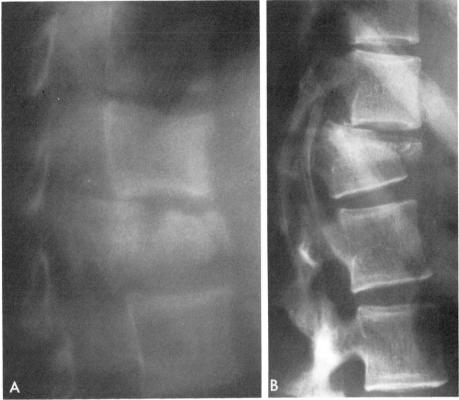

**Figure 2–17.** Comminution and displacement of the posterior cortex of the vertebral body *(A)* as well as vertebral body displacement *(B)* are specific radiographic changes which should be sought and commented upon.

tex *of the vertebral body,* and *vertebral body displacement* (Fig. 2–17). Specific signs indicating posterior spinal column injury and hence allowing the radiologist to appreciate the potential for acute instability of the spine include *fracture through the neural arch* or *posterior elements, widening of the interpediculate distance,* and *discontinuity of the spinous process* (Fig. 2–18) (Table 2–1).[15, 16] *Paravertebral soft tissue swelling* due to paraspinal hematoma indicates acute trauma and helps indicate whether bony changes

**Table 2–1.** IMPORTANT RADIOGRAPHIC FINDINGS OF TRAUMA TO THE SPINE

Comminution
Displacement of the posterior cortex of the vertebral body
Vertebral body displacement
Fracture through the neural arch or posterior elements
Widening of the interpediculate distance
Discontinuity of the spinous process
Paravertebral soft tissue swelling

such as anterior wedging of the vertebral bodies are acute or remote (Fig. 2–19).

*Myelography* is not routinely indicated but may be useful in patients who have neurologic damage without obvious skeletal damage, or in those whose level of neurologic damage does not correspond with the level of skeletal damage, and in those experiencing progressive neurologic deficit after stabilization of the spine.[1] It is useful in demonstrating degree of cord compression, especially by soft tissue structures such as hematoma and extruded disc material which are not radiodense and cannot be appreciated by conventional radiography. Compression secondary to bony fragments, however, is best demonstrated by computed tomography.

Prior to CT scanning, gas myelography furnished more information about the spinal cord and its relationship to the spinal canal than oil myelography, allowing demonstration of spinal cord swelling, and obviating the fear of blood mixing with oily contrast

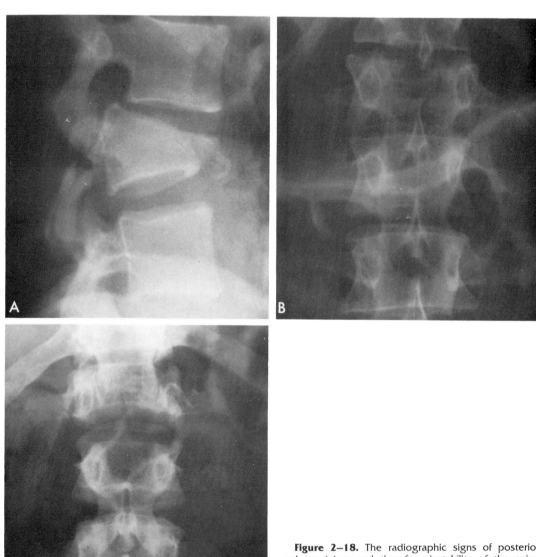

**Figure 2–18.** The radiographic signs of posterior column injury and therefore instability of the spine include (A) fracture through the neural arch or posterior elements, (B) widening of the interpediculate distance and (C) discontinuity of the spinous process.

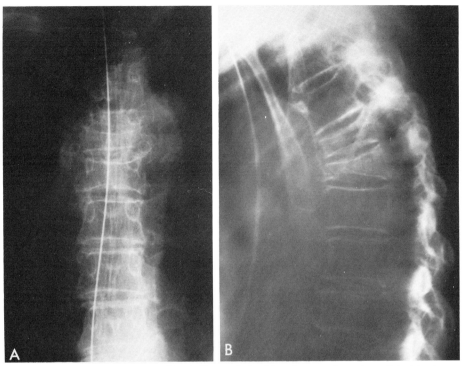

**Figure 2–19.** Paravertebral soft tissue swelling indicates that mid and upper thoracic vertebral body compression fractures are acute.

medium in the spinal canal. Since it was performed in combination with tomography and bony analysis was also obtained at the same time, however, a multidirectional poly-tome was mandatory for this examination. More recently, water soluble contrast media (metrizamide) has been found superior to gas myelography (Fig. 2–20). At present, however, computed tomography (Fig. 2–21) is probably replacing the myelogram because it can demonstrate hematoma, disc, or bony encroachment upon the spinal canal using the computed radiograph or reformatted sagittal or coronal images to localize the level studied.[17, 18, 19, 20, 21] At present, CT scanning has probably replaced polytomography in the evaluation and further delineation of fractures of the thoracolumbar spine because of the additional information yielded.

**Treatment**

Although treatment is not an obvious concern of the radiologist, the diagnostician should have an appreciation of the influence of the radiographic findings in association with the clinical findings on the subsequent management of the patient. As in many other areas of medicine, the treatment of spinal fractures has evolved and changed over the years and is predominantly influenced by the presence or absence of neurologic damage and whether the injury is stable or unstable. *Stable injuries without neurologic damage* include anterior wedge, lateral wedge, and compression fractures, which require bed rest and perhaps a brace or body jacket. *Stable injuries with neurologic deficit* result from compression of the spinal cord or nerve roots rather than motion at the fracture site. If neurologic deficit is complete for 48 hours, surgical decompression generally will not restore lost neurologic function. On the other hand, incomplete neurologic loss or compression of the cauda equina may benefit from decompression in the form of reduction with or without a limited laminectomy. *Unstable injuries without neurologic deficit* necessitate open reduction in association with internal fixation and spinal fusion.[2] Reduction will usually accomplish decompression, which has been used since at least the fifth century B. C., although the

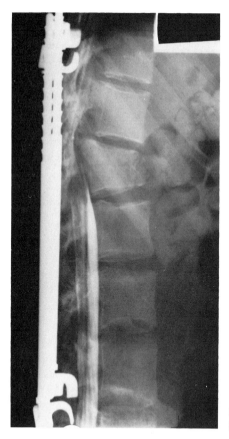

**Figure 2–20.** Water-soluble contrast media myelogram demonstrates a high-grade block in a patient with progressive neurologic deficit after stabilization of the spine.

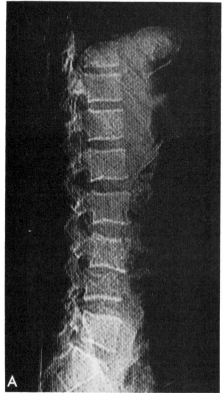

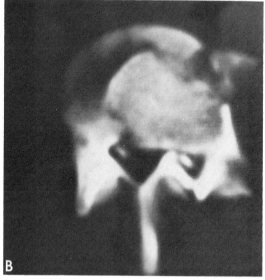

**Figure 2–21.** A computed radiograph in the lateral projection demonstrates fractures of L-3 and L-4 with retrolisthesis of L-4 *(A)*. *B*, A transverse scan through L-4 demonstrates a comminuted fracture of the vertebral body with displacement of a large major fragment into the canal as well as several loose fragments in the canal.

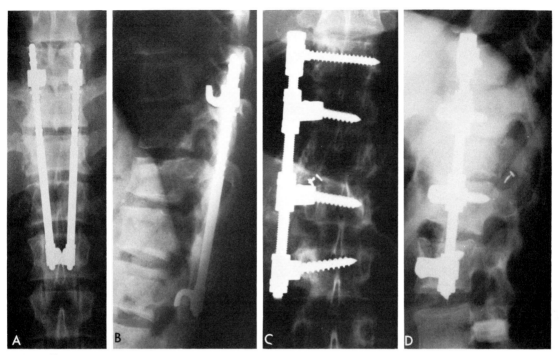

**Figure 2–22.** Posterior (Harrington) (*A* and *B*) and anterior (Dunn) (*C* and *D*) rod fixation of the spine.

actual method has changed somewhat. Basically, the fixation device employed in stabilization of the spine may be a posterior (Harrington) or anterior (Dunn) rod (Fig. 2–22). The brackets of the Harrington rod are placed in distraction or compression and fit over the lamina in the lumbar spine and over the pedicle in the thoracic spine (since there is not enough room to fit over the lamina in the thoracic spine). The brackets should ideally be two vertebrae above and two below the level of the fracture. The screws of the Dunn rod are placed directly into the vertebral body. There should be no change in position or alignment of the fixation device on interval radiographs (Fig. 2–23). A concomitant spinal fusion is performed to ensure stabilization and the graft bone for the fusion loses its granular appearance and becomes solid as it is incorporated into the spine (Fig. 2–24).

*Slippage of the brackets* may occur and evidence of this obtained on the anteroposterior or lateral view. Oblique projections are very useful in confirming slippage by showing the brackets to lie definitely outside of the spine (Fig. 2–25). *Progressive kyphosis* may occur and is readily observed and measured on the lateral projection (Fig. 2–26). This may be associated with increased vertebral body compression due to failure of rigid fixation or failure of fusion.

*Failure of fusion* may cause persistent and progressive back pain. Linear or computed tomography may be effective in demonstrating this failure of fusion or pseudarthrosis (Fig. 2–27). *Postsurgical infection* may occur, resulting in progressive increased pain and bony destruction.

## DISC DISEASE

The diagnosis of disc disease made on a clinical basis has been dependent upon myelography in the past for confirmation. Computed tomography, however, has provided a noninvasive means of visualizing both the bone and soft tissue structures of the spine and has allowed demonstration of bulging and herniated discs as well as facet joint disease (Fig. 2–28). In addition, computed tomography has been helpful in the evaluation of the postoperative back patient with recurrent symptoms due to spinal nerve compression and spinal canal stenosis, resulting from posterolateral fusion overgrowth (Fig. 2–29).[22–26]

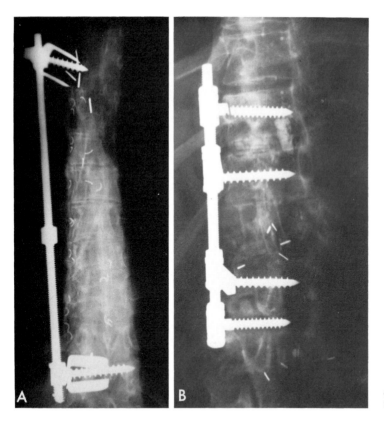

**Figure 2–23.** Pulling out of screw and bracket of Dunn rod *(A)* and fracture of screw *(B)*.

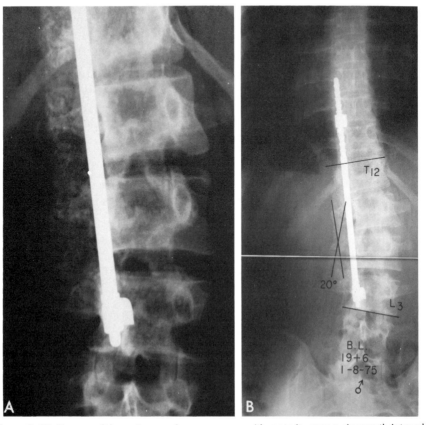

**Figure 2–24.** Bone graft loses its granular appearance with maturity over a six-month interval.

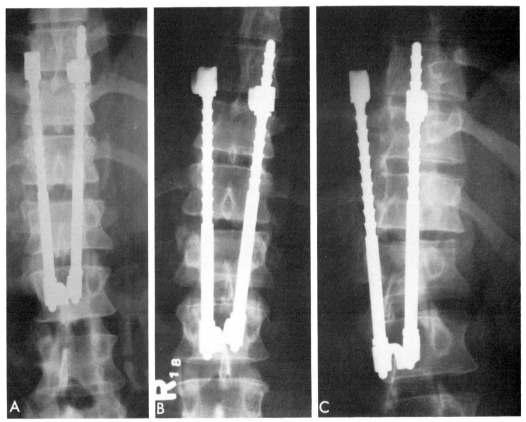

**Figure 2–25.** Interval disengagement of the right superior bracket is noted between the two anteroposterior projections (*A* and *B*) and confirmed on the oblique projection *(C)*.

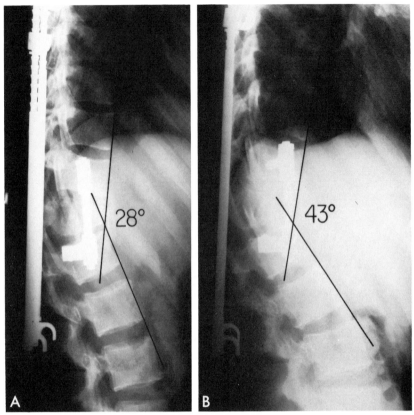

**Figure 2–26.** Failure of stabilization of the spine by both posterior (Harrington) and anterior (Dunn) rod fixation causes a progressive increase in kyphosis from 28 to 43 degrees. Note disengagement of the inferior Harrington rod brackets.

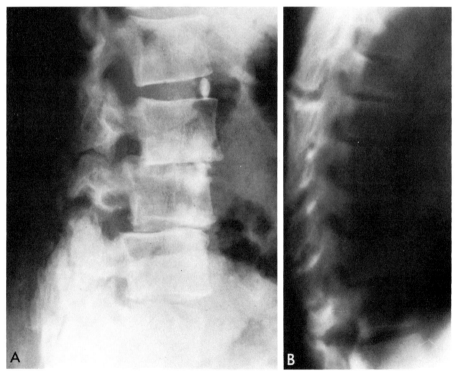

**Figure 2–27.** *A,* Failure of fusion may result in a pseudarthrosis and pain. *B,* Tomography is effective in demonstrating the lucent cleft and sclerosis associated with pseudarthrosis. Note, multiple pseudarthroses (different patient from *A*).

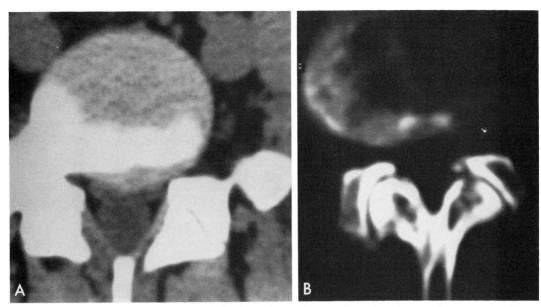

**Figure 2–28.** CT scans demonstrate central disc herniation and encroachment on the spinal nerve root exiting on the left *(A)* and facet joint degenerative disease *(B)*.

## SPINAL FUSION

Spinal fusion is performed following fracture dislocation as well as in the treatment of disc disease, spondylolisthesis, and scoliosis. The fusion may be posterolateral and involve the transverse processes or anterior in location. The bone graft providing the fusion should gradually mature and be in-

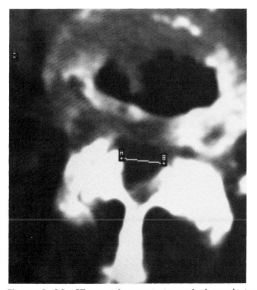

**Figure 2–29.** CT scan demonstrates spinal canal stenosis resulting from posterolateral fusion overgrowth.

corporated into a solid fusion mass. This is indicated radiographically by the loss of distinct margins and outlines of the individual bone graft fragments (Fig. 2–30).

A *pseudarthrosis* may develop, allowing motion at the fusion site, and be the cause of persistent back pain following a spinal fusion. This is observed radiographically as a radiolucent cleft in the fusion mass, frequently with sclerotic borders. Lateral bending films made in the anteroposterior projection or flexion-extension films made in the lateral projection may delineate this cleft to better advantage by causing distraction at the site of pseudarthrosis, but these are not always diagnostic (Fig. 2–31). In addition, flexion and extension films made in the lateral projection with the patient erect may show motion at the fusion site. It is important to note, however, that an apparent pseudarthrosis may acutally represent fibrous union and that an actual pseudarthrosis along with motion at the fusion site may not be associated with pain.[27] Epstein,[28] on the other hand, has noted these maneuvers are of doubtful reliability. We have found polytomography in the lateral or oblique projection, depending on the plain film projection in which the fusion is best visualized, to demonstrate effectively a pseudarthrosis if one is present.

*Postfusion spinal stenosis* due to over-

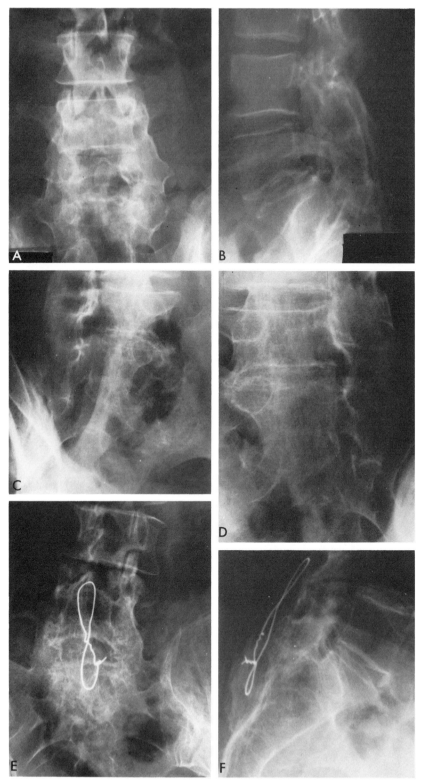

**Figure 2–30.** Posterolateral spinal fusion without wire stabilization. *A* to *D,* Bony fusion mass is solid and intact, and oblique projections are useful in demonstrating this. *E* and *F,* Posterolateral spinal fusion with wire stabilization.

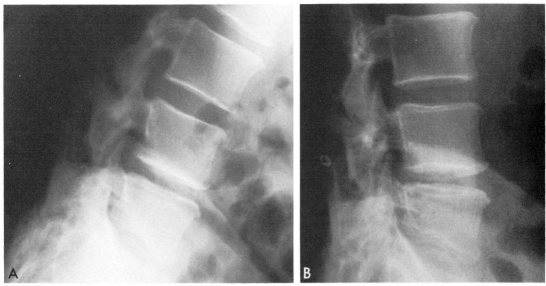

**Figure 2–31.** Flexion-extension series demonstrates separation at the sites of pseudarthroses at the L-3 to L-4 and L-4 to L-5 levels on flexion *(A)*.

growth of the fusion may also cause persistent postoperative back pain. This spinal canal compromise is usually not demonstrated by routine radiography but may be well delineated by computed tomography and is probably a more common cause of postfusion back pain than has been realized in the past[29, 30] (see Fig. 2–29).

*Infection*, postlaminectomy or postfusion, may cause destruction of the corresponding disc space, vertebral end plates, and vertebral bodies. Irregularity of the endplates, narrowing of the disc space due to disc destruction, and vertebral body sclerosis are the radiographic changes indicating infection (Fig. 2–32). *Needle aspiration* of the involved area may help in isolating and identifying the organism.

When a laminectomy is performed without stabilization by a fusion, the laminectomy may be so excessive that an iatrogenic spondylolisthesis results (Fig. 2–33).

## SCOLIOSIS

Scoliosis is a lateral curvature of the spine with varying degrees of rotation of the vertebral bodies around a vertical axis. Although many different classifications of scoliosis have been proposed, a more simple scheme divides the scoliotic curve into the nonstructural and the structural varieties.

The *nonstructural* curve is a flexible curve which corrects with the patient bending towards the convex side. An example of this type of curve is that associated with a leg length discrepancy where the pelvis is tilted downward on the short side. The *structural scoliotic curve* is a rigid curve that fails to correct with the patient bending towards the convex side. This category includes *idiopathic scoliosis, congenital scoliosis,* and *neuromuscular scoliosis* caused by diseases such as poliomyelitis or muscular dystrophy (Fig. 2–34).

*Idiopathic scoliosis,* the most common type of scoliosis observed by both the radiologist and orthopedic surgeon, is hereditary. This type of scoliosis exhibits several different curve patterns, the most common of which is the *right thoracic curve,* which is the *major* or *structural curve* in association with an adjacent curve that goes in the opposite direction and is referred to as the *secondary, compensatory,* or *minor curve.* Less common major curve patterns include the *thoracolumbar curve,* convex to the right or left, *the double major curve,* consisting of two structural or major curves such as a right thoracic and left lumbar curve, and a *lumbar major curve,* usually convex to the left (Fig. 2–35).

*Congenital scoliosis* may be classified as *vertebral* or *extravertebral curves.* The vertebral curves are characterized by congenital

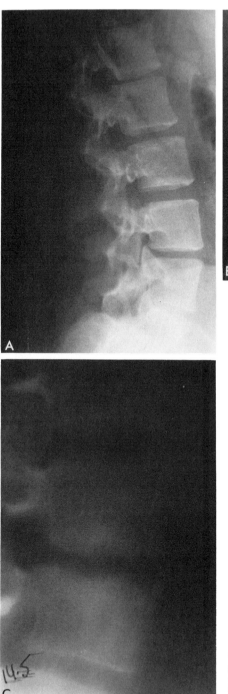

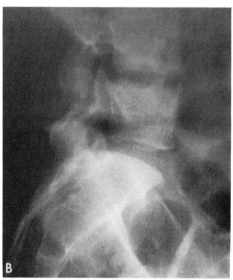

**Figure 2–32.** Postoperative disc space infection is indicated by rapid narrowing of the disc space and vertebral end-plate destruction (A) prior to laminectomy. B and C, Plain film and tomogram demonstrating postlaminectomy disc space infection.

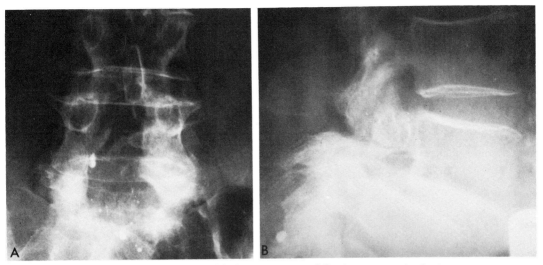

**Figure 2–33.** Iatrogenic spondylolisthesis may occur following an excessive laminectomy.

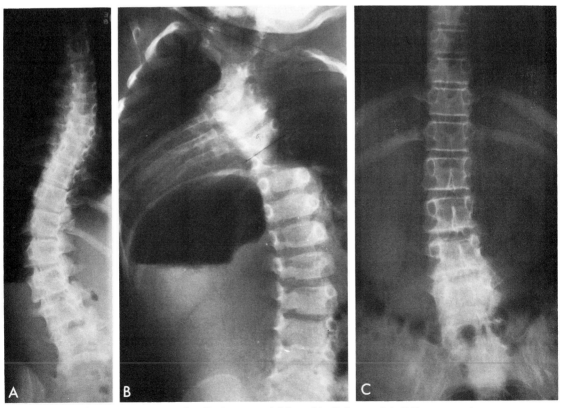

**Figure 2–34.** Types of scoliosis curves: *A*, Idiopathic. *B*, Congenital. *C*, Neuromuscular.

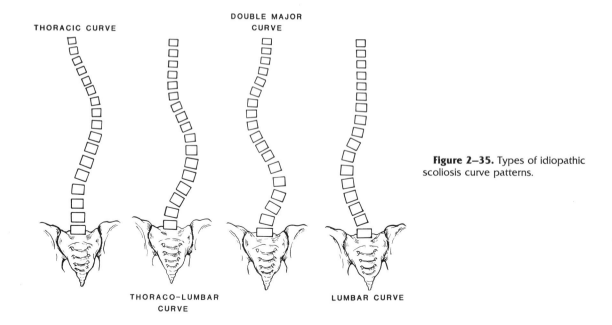

THORACIC CURVE

DOUBLE MAJOR CURVE

**Figure 2–35.** Types of idiopathic scoliosis curve patterns.

THORACO–LUMBAR CURVE

LUMBAR CURVE

vertebral anomalies such as myelomeningocele, wedge vertebrae, hemivertebrae, congenital bars, and block vertebrae. The extravertebral curves are associated with congenital anomalies outside the vertebral bodies, such as congenital rib fusions (Fig. 2–34).[31]

### Radiographic Evaluation of the Preoperative Scoliosis Patient

The preoperative scoliosis patient is evaluated with *erect anteroposterior and lateral views* of the spine from the occiput to the sacrum and a spot lateral view of the lumbosacral junction to demonstrate spondylolysis and spondylolisthesis. A standard scoliosis film cassette makes it possible to fit the entire spine on the film. *Right and left side bending films in recumbency* are obtained to distinguish structural (fixed angulation) from nonstructural curves as well as to determine the degree of flexibility and suppleness of the ligaments and associated soft tissue structures. These films provide an idea of the extent of correctability of the primary curve. Pelvic tilt in the erect position suggests probable leg length discrepancy, and sitting films will help eliminate this discrepancy. When scoliosis is associated with neuromuscular disease (cerebral

palsy, polio), a pelvic tilt is also frequently observed. The question of whether the scoliosis and pelvic tilt are secondary to hip muscle contracture, causing a nonstructural curve benefitting by release of the muscle contractures, or whether the scoliotic curve is structural arises. If the curve reduces with wooden blocks placed under the buttock on the convex side of the curve, it is nonstructural, and release of the hip contractures will improve the scoliosis.[32]

### Measurement of the Curve

The *Cobb method* is recognized as the method of choice for curve measurement by the Scoliosis Research Society. It is based on determining the *transitional vertebra* at the top and bottom of each curve. The transitional vertebra is the one at either end of the curve which tilts the greatest toward the concavity of the curve. The measurement should be made from the superior border of the superior transitional vertebra to the inferior border of the inferior transitional vertebra. Horizontal lines are drawn through these landmarks and a perpendicular line is then drawn to each horizontal line and the intersecting angles measured (Fig. 2–36). If the vertebral end plates are not sufficiently distinct to draw the horizontal line, then the

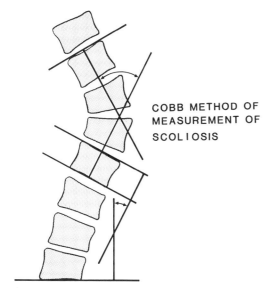

**Figure 2–36.** The Cobb method is recognized by the Scoliosis Research Society as the method of choice in measuring the scoliotic curve.

pedicles are utilized. The curve is described according to the side of the convexity at the level of the deformity.[31]

*Rotation* of the vertebral bodies within the measured curve can be assessed on the anteroposterior radiograph by the amount of midline shift of one of the pedicles toward a vertical axis. By convention, this is graded from zero rotation through 4 + (Fig. 2–37).

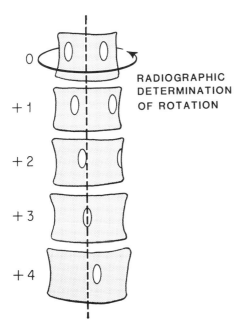

**Figure 2–37.** Radiographic determination of rotation.

Rotation determines the extent of required bone fusion and the rigidity of the curve.[33]

*Skeletal maturation* is an important factor in the treatment of scoliosis and can be assessed on the radiograph. The iliac crest apophyses fuse approximately three to six months before the ring apophyses of the vertebral body; therefore, three to six months after closure of the iliac crest apophyses spinal growth ceases. At this time no added benefit will be obtained from a brace and, if necessary, surgery may be performed.

**Treatment**

The main reason for treatment of scoliosis is to prevent progression of the curve, since impairment of cardiopulmonary function may occur with curves greater than 60 degrees. With respect to progression, if the scoliotic curve is less than 20 degrees before spinal growth ceases it probably will not progress. If the curve is 40 degrees it probably will increase, and if between 20 and 40 degrees it may or may not increase.

The two methods of treatment of scoliosis are spinal bracing with exercises or surgery. Surgery is performed when bracing is ineffective. The surgical approach may be *anterior*, utilizing a *Dwyer cable*, or *posterior*, utlilizing a *Harrington rod*.

*Anterior approach.* Screws are inserted into each vertebral body and a wire along the convex side of the curve is wrapped around each screw. The intervertebral discs are removed between the vertebrae in the curve, and traction is applied to the wire, allowing correction of the curve (Fig. 2–38).

*Posterior approach.* This approach is more commonly employed and utilizes Harrington rod instrumentation to maintain correction of the curve and bony fusion. The laminae and spinous processes are decorticated and the posterior facet joints obliterated. An autogenous bone graft taken from the iliac crest is applied along the concave side of the curve to be fused. Usually the fusion area incorporates one vertebral body above the superior transitional vertebra and two vertebral bodies below the inferior transitional vertebra as well as all rotated vertebrae. Lack of incorporation of the rotated vertebrae in the spinal fusion may cause progression of the curve.

The Harrington rod, utilized as a distrac-

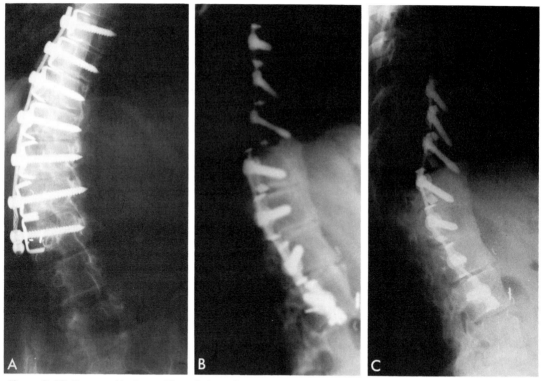

**Figure 2–38.** Dwyer cable. Interval lateral views demonstrate incorporation of bone graft and fusion of intervertebral disc spaces.

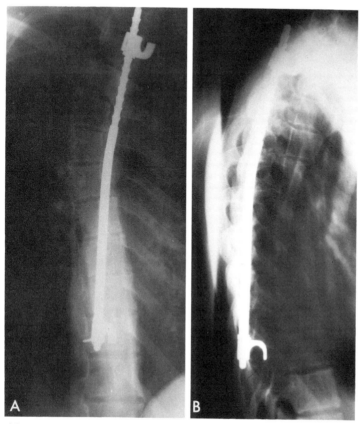

**Figure 2–39.** Harrington rod with normal bowing to accommodate scoliotic *(A)*, and kyphotic *(B)* curves.

tion rod, is inserted on the concave side of the curve with the superior bracket engaged on the pedicle of the thoracic vertebra and the inferior bracket engaged on the lamina of the lumbar vertebra (Fig. 2–39). At times, an additional rod is utilized in compression along the convex side of the curve (interconnecting rod) (Fig. 2–40).

## Radiologic Evaluation of the Postoperative Scoliosis Patient

The goal of rod instrumentation is to achieve approximately 50 per cent correction of the scoliotic curve. The bony fusion usually becomes solid by the ninth postoperative month and is best evaluated on 60-degree supine oblique projections.[34] When the Dwyer cable has been used, the disc spaces should become obliterated. Progression of the curve postoperatively may be due to failure of incorporating the rotated vertebrae in the spinal fusion, pseudarthrosis, slippage of the brackets, or fracture of the rod or cable (Fig. 2–41).[35] *Erect anteroposterior* and *lateral views* are obtained at interval follow-up examinations to measure and compare the curve. Smaller films than

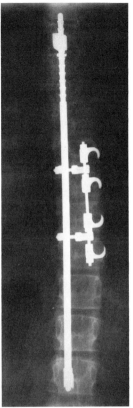

**Figure 2–40.** Harrington and interconnecting rods.

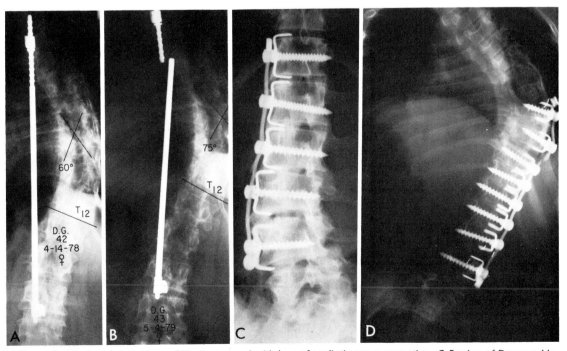

**Figure 2–41.** *A* and *B*, Fracture of Harrington rod with loss of scoliotic curve correction. *C*, Fraying of Dwyer cable. *D*, Fracture of Dwyer cable.

the standard scoliosis cassette may be used as long as the entire extent of the surgical scar will fit on the film. *Tomography* may be helpful in demonstrating a pseudarthrosis when this is suspected. A normal loss of correction may occur postoperatively, up to 11 per cent of the original correction[36] or 10 degrees or less.[34]

## Kyphosis

The kyphotic curve in the thoracic spine is normally 10 to 20 degrees and the lordotic curve in the lumbar spine is normally 15 to 20 degrees.[37] Abnormal kyphotic deformity in the thoracic spine may result from Scheuermann's disease or be associated with scoliosis. Kyphosis greater than 40 degrees is considered abnormal in the thoracic spine and is measured by drawing lines tangential to the end plates of the proximal and distal end vertebrae, drawing perpendiculars to these lines, and measuring the angle between the two intersecting perpendiculars (Fig. 2–42). The end vertebrae are those most tilted from the horizontal.[38] Anterior instrumentation may be utilized to correct a significant kyphotic deformity.

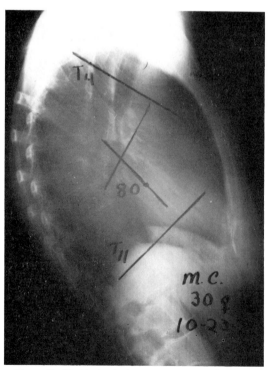

**Figure 2–42.** Method of measurement of kyphosis.

## References

1. Rockwood CA, Green DP: Fractures. Vol. 2. Philadelphia, JB Lippincott, 1975, pp 816–903
2. Bradford DS, Thompson RC: Fractures and dislocations of the spine, indications for surgical intervention. Minnesota Medicine 59:711–720, 1976
3. Koreska J, Robertson D, Mills RH, Gibson DA, Albiser AM: Biomechanics of the lumbar spine and its clinical significance. Orthop Clin N Am 8:121–133, 1977
4. Burke DC, Murray DD: The management of thoracic and thoraco-lumbar injuries of the spine with neurological involvement. J Bone Joint Surg 48B:72–78, 1976
5. Holdsworth FW: Fractures, dislocations, and fracture-dislocations of the spine. J Bone Joint Surg 45B:6–20, 1963
6. Huelke DF, Kaufer H: Vertebral column injuries and seat belts. J Trauma 15:304–318, 1975
7. Fletcher BD, Brogdon BG: Seat belt fractures of the spine and sternum. JAMA 200:177–178, 1967
8. Carroll TB, Gruber FH: Seat belt fractures, a report of two cases. Radiology 91:517–518, 1968
9. Smith WS, Kaufer H: Patterns and mechanisms of lumbar injuries associated with lap seat belts. J Bone Joint Surg 51A:239–254, 1969
10. Gelman MI, Umber JS: Fractures of the thoracolumbar spine in ankylosing spondylitis. AJR 130:485–491, 1978
11. Hanafee W, Crandall P: Trauma of the spine and its contents. Radiol Clin N Am 12:365–382, 1966
12. Calenoff L, Chessare JW, Rogers LF, Roerge J, Rosen JS: Multiple level spinal injuries, importance of early recognition. AJR 130:665–669, 1978
13. Rogers LF, Thayer C, Weinberg PE, Kim KS: Acute injuries of the upper thoracic spine associated with paraplegia. AJNR 1:89–95, 1980
14. Kaufer H, Hayes JT: Lumbar fracture—dislocation, a study of twenty-one cases. J Bone Joint Surg 48A:712–730, 1966
15. Quesada RS, Greenbaum EI, Hertl A, Zoda F: Widened interpedicular distance secondary to trauma. J Trauma 15:167–169, 1975
16. Chiroff RT, Sachs GL: Discontinuity of the spinous process on standard roentgenographs as an aid in the diagnosis of unstable fractures of the spine. J Trauma 16:313–316, 1976
17. Laasonen EM: Myelography for severe thoracolumbar injuries. Neuroradiology 13:165–168, 1977
18. Pay NT, George AE, Benjamin MV, Bergeron RT, Lin JP, Kricheff II: Positive and negative contrast meylography in spinal trauma. Radiology 123:103–111, 1977
19. Tadmor R, Davis KR, Roberson GH, New PJF, Taveras JM: Computed tomographic evaluation of traumatic spinal injuries. Radiology 127:825–827, 1978
20. Colley DP, Dunsker SB: Traumatic narrowing of the dorsolumbar spinal canal demonstrated by computed tomography. Radiology 129:95–98, 1978
21. Glenn WV, Rhodes ML, Altschuler EM, Wiltse CC, et al.: Multiplanar display computerized body tomography applications in the lumbar spine. Spine 4:282–352, 1979
22. Glenn WV, Rhodes ML, Altschuler EM, Wiltse CC, Kostanek C, Kuo YM: Multiplanar display computerized body tomography applications in the lumbar spine. Spine 4:282–352, 1979

23. Burton CV, Heithoff KB, Kirkaldz-Willis W, Raz DC: Computed tomographic scanning and the lumbar spine. Part II: Clinical considerations. Spine 4:356–368, 1979
24. Carrera GF, Haughton VM, Syvertsen A, Williams AL: Computed tomography of the lumbar facet joints. Radiology 134:145–148, 1980
25. Haughton VM, Syvertsen A, Williams AL: Soft tissue anatomy within the spinal canal as seen in computed tomography. Radiology 134:649–655, 1980
26. Williams AL, Haughton VM, Syvertsen A: Computed tomography in the diagnosis of herniated nucleus pulposus. Radiology 135:95–99, 1980
27. Lettin AWF: Diagnosis and treatment of lumbar instability. J Bone Joint Surg 49:520–29, 1967
28. Epstein BS: The Spine, a Radiological Text and Atlas. 4th edition. Philadelphia, Lea and Febiger, 1976, p 607
29. Quencer RM, Murtagh FR, Post MJ, Rosomof HL, Stokes NA: Postoperative bony stenosis of the lumbar spinal canal: evaluation of 164 symptomatic patients with axial radiography. AJR 131:1059–1064, 1978
30. Sheldon JJ, Sersland T, Leborgne J: Computed tomography of the lower lumbar vertebral column. Normal anatomy and the stenotic canal. Radiology 124:113–118, 1977
31. Klein HA: Scoliosis. Ciba Clinical Symposia Vol. 30, Number 1, 1978
32. Dunn H: Personal communication
33. McAlister WH, Shackelford GD: Measurement of spinal curvature. Radiol Clin N Am 13:113–121, 1975
34. Goldstein LA: The surgical management of scoliosis. Clin Orthop 35:95–115, 1964
35. Wilkinson RH, Willi UV, Gilsanz V, Mulrihill D: Radiographic evaluation of the spine after surgical correction of scoliosis. AJR 133:703–709, 1979
36. Fowles JV, Drummond DS, L'Ecuyer S, Roy L, Kassab M: Untreated scoliosis in the adult. Clin Orthop Rel Res 134:212–217, 1978
37. Hoppenfeld S: Scoliosis. A Manual of Concept and Treatment. Philadelphia, JB Lippincott, 1967
38. McAlister WH, Shackelford GD: Classification of spinal curvatures. Radiol Clin N Am 13:93–112, 1975

# 3

# THE UPPER EXTREMITY: SHOULDER, HUMERUS, ELBOW, AND FOREARM

## DISORDERS OF THE SHOULDER

The painful shoulder requiring orthopedic attention usually results from a degenerative or post-traumatic process. The rotator cuff, which represents a common musculotendinous insertion of the supraspinatus, infraspinatus, teres minor, and subscapularis muscles with the shoulder joint capsule, may undergo degeneration with advancing age.

### Calcific Tendonitis

Calcification may occur in the area of degeneration, usually the supraspinatus tendon, resulting in a calcific tendonitis with associated inflammation of the overlying bursa and subsequent bursitis. Internal and external rotation views are helpful in demonstrating these deposits (Fig. 3–1).

### Rotator Cuff Tear

Degeneration of the rotator cuff may result in a tear, which may also occur following trauma. Plain film changes resulting from a chronic rotator cuff tear include reduction in the distance between the convexity of the humeral head and the undersurface of the acromion process, mechanical erosion of the undersurface of the acromion process with resulting concavity, and cystic and sclerotic changes in the greater tuberosity; however,

arthrography is needed for confirmation (Fig. 3–2).[1] These changes may also be observed in rheumatoid arthritis and are probably, at least in part, due to an associated rotator cuff tear. Since surgical repair involves the soft tissues, no specific postsurgical changes are seen on the postoperative films.

**Shoulder Arthrography.** Shoulder arthrography is most commonly utilized in demonstrating the presence of a rotator cuff tear. Single or double contrast technique may be used.[2, 3] With either method, however, the presence of contrast medium in the subacromial-subdeltoid bursa confirms the presence of a tear (Fig. 3–3). Occasionally, contrast medium will enter the acromioclavicular joint during a shoulder arthrogram in the presence of an extensive chronic degenerative rotator cuff tear, probably owing to disruption of the acromioclavicular joint capsule (Fig. 3–4).[4] Other entities that may be sources of shoulder pain and may be diagnosed by arthrography include adhesive capsulitis, rupture of the long head of the biceps muscle, loose bodies, and synovial cysts (Fig. 3–5). More recently, shoulder arthrography employing a greater volume of contrast medium has been described as a nonoperative modality in the treatment of adhesive capsulitis, implementing positive long-term results.[5]

### Recurrent Dislocation of the Shoulder

Recurrent dislocation of the shoulder may result from a variety of factors, including

44

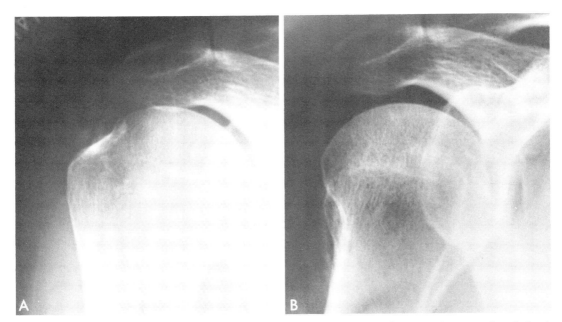

**Figure 3–1.** *A,* External rotation view demonstrates calcium deposition within the supraspinatus tendon. *B,* On the internal rotation view the calcium is obscured by the bone.

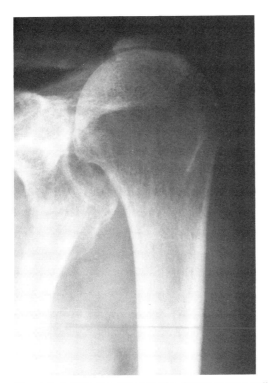

**Figure 3–2.** Plain film changes of a chronic rotator cuff tear include cephalad migration of the humeral head and erosion of the undersurface of the acromion process.

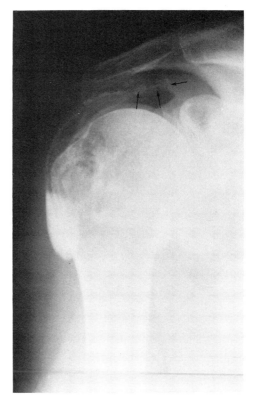

**Figure 3–3.** Arthrographic demonstration of a rotator cuff tear. A double contrast examination demonstrates filling of the subacromial-subdeltoid bursa, indicating a rotator cuff tear. The torn fragmented rotator cuff is well visualized (arrows).

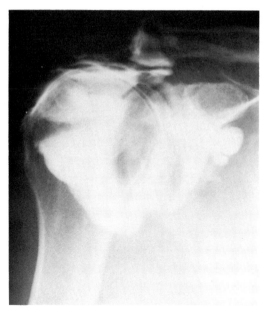

**Figure 3–4.** Arthrogram (single contrast) demonstrates a rotator cuff tear as well as disruption of the acromioclavicular joint capsule indicated by contrast medium filling the subacromial-subdeltoid bursa and the acromioclavicular joint.

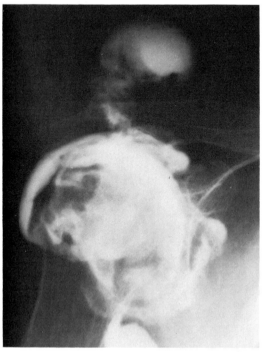

**Figure 3–5.** Arthrogram demonstrates a synovial cyst communicating with the joint space.

inadequate immobilization or disruption of the cartilaginous labrum and its capsular attachment after the initial dislocation. It also appears to be age-related, in that it occurs much more frequently in patients under 20 years of age.[11] An accentuated groove-like defect or a notch in the posterolateral aspect of the humeral head, best seen on an internal rotation view or axillary lateral projection, is a radiographic sign of previous anterior dislocation and is referred to as the Hill-Sachs deformity. This defect may consist of localized flattening of the humeral head, a wedge-shaped defect, or a linear indentation of bone running parallel to the humeral shaft (Fig. 3–6).[12, 13] It represents an impaction fracture at the point where the posterior surface of the humeral head hits the glenoid process. (A similar defect may occur on the anteromedial surface of the humeral head in a posterior dislocation). Associated capsular laxity allowing recurrent dislocation may occur, necessitating surgical repair. Many procedures have been devised to correct this laxity, having as a common theme tightening of the capsule as well as additional reinforcement provided by muscle tendon transfer. Since this involves primarily soft tissue repair, few radiographic changes are appreciated, other than the presence of metallic staples or screws. Comparison of staple or screw position on successive films may reveal a change, indicating a loss of the tethering effect and possible failure of the procedure. Fracture through the staple or screw may also occur, with subsequent migration of the metallic fragments.

**Surgical Repair for Recurrent Dislocation.** The Putti-Platt procedure consists of shortening and reinforcing the capsule and subscapularis muscle.[14]

The Bankart procedure is a reattachment of the capsule and labrum to the glenoid rim and is often done in association with the Putti-Platt procedure to ensure greater stability of the shoulder (staples are used)[15] (Fig. 3–7).

The Magnuson-Stack procedure consists of transferring the subscapularis muscle insertion from the lesser tuberosity laterally to the greater tuberosity to increase stability.[16, 17]

A modified Bristow procedure, also called the anterior bone block operation, consists of transferring the coracoid process with its

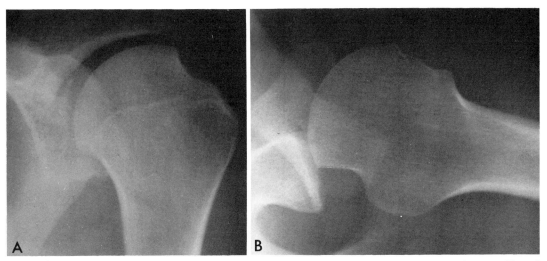

**Figure 3—6.** The Hill-Sachs deformity represents an impaction fracture and indicates previous dislocation. Note the groove-like defect on the lateral and posterior aspects of the humeral head.

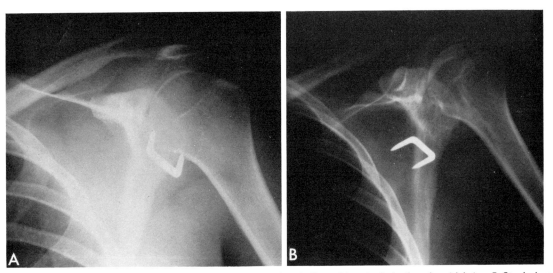

**Figure 3—7.** *A,* A Bankart procedure has been performed as indicated by staple in the glenoidal rim. *B,* Staple has subsequently loosened and migrated.

attached conjoined tendon (coracobrachialis and short head of the biceps muscles) to the anterior rim of the glenoid. The bone block impedes anterior dislocation, whereas the conjoined tendon reinforces the joint capsule. This procedure is recognized radiographically by screw fixation of the coracoid process to the inferior glenoid rim and may be complicated by a break in the screw, nonunion of the coracoid process, or migration of the bone block or screw (Fig. 3–8). Resorption of bone around the screw evidently does not indicate loosening or failure of the procedure.[18]

Staple capsulorrhaphy consists of tightening the joint capsule by stapling it directly to the bone. Muscles are not detached, shortened, or transplanted. The staples may break or loosen. Each staple is implanted into the neck of the scapula approximately parallel

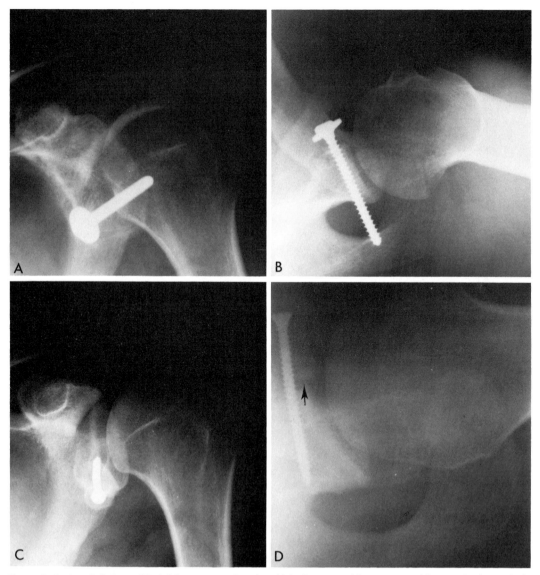

**Figure 3–8.** A and B, A modified Bristow procedure in which the corocoid process and its attached muscle have been transferred to the anterior rim of the glenoid is indicated by the presence of a screw in the inferior rim of the glenoid. C and D, Nonunion of transplanted corocoid process to anterior glenoid process (arrow).

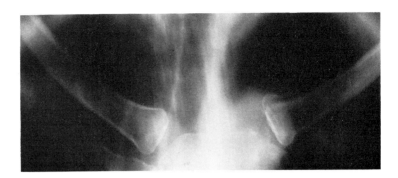

**Figure 3–9.** Tomography is useful in demonstrating and confirming fractures of the head of the clavicle.

to the surface of the glenoid cavity and 5 to 8 mm from the articular surface. The staple should not penetrate into the glenoid cavity.

## DISORDERS OF THE CLAVICLE

### Fracture of the Clavicle

Fractures of the clavicle may involve the inner, middle, or outer third of the clavicle and may be well demonstrated by an anteroposterior projection with the tube angled 45 degrees cephalad. Fractures of the head of the clavicle may require tomography for confirmation (Fig. 3–9). Complications such as malunion may occur, but nonunion is rare. Post-traumatic arthritis of the acromioclavicular or sternoclavicular joint or resorption of the distal end of the clavicle may occur, which is painful, necessitating excision of the distal or medial end of the clavicle.[19–23]

### Acromioclavicular Joint Disease

Trauma to the acromioclavicular joint, manifested by widening or separation of the joint or elevation of the distal clavicle, may be treated by slings or internal fixation using wires, which may break.

Surgical resection of the distal end of the clavicle may be performed to alleviate painful post-traumatic or degenerative arthritis or rheumatoid arthritis (Fig. 3–10). At times postsurgical changes in the distal clavicle are difficult to distinguish from the resorptive changes occurring in rheumatoid arthritis, although rheumatoid arthritis usually causes a tapered appearance (Fig. 3–11).

### Disruption of the Acromioclavicular Joint

The normal width of the acromioclavicular joint is maintained by the acromiocla-

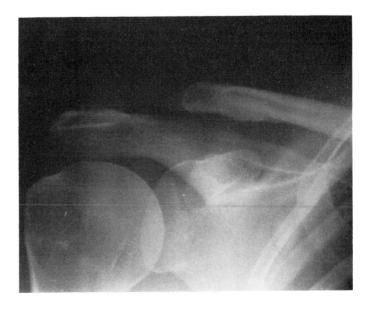

**Figure 3–10.** Surgical resection of the distal end of the clavicle may be performed in the treatment of post-traumatic or degenerative arthritis as well as rheumatoid arthritis of the acromioclavicular joint.

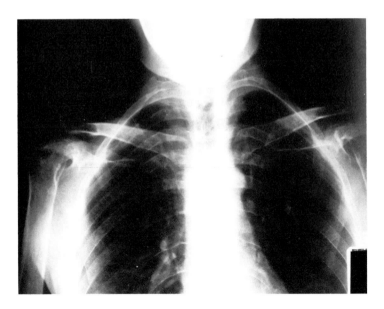

**Figure 3–11.** Rheumatoid arthritis usually causes a tapered appearance of the distal clavicle in association with erosive changes in the shoulder joints and deossification.

vicular ligaments, whereas the clavicle is maintained at a normal level with the acromion process by the coracoclavicular ligament. The normal distance between the coracoid process and the clavicle may vary from 1.1 to 1.3 cm.[24, 25]

Acromioclavicular joint disruption is classified radiologically into three types in order to describe the extent of injury as well as to establish a basis for treatment. Stress views are important, since they assess the true extent of the injury. At times, acromioclavic-

ular separation may be demonstrated on erect films of the shoulder when no separation is suspected, and therefore radiographs of the shoulder should be obtained erect in cases of suspected trauma whenever possible (Fig. 3–12). A Type I injury shows no radiographic abnormality. A Type II injury shows minimal elevation of the clavicle or widening of the acromioclavicular joint due to disruption of the acromioclavicular ligament, or both (Fig. 3–13). Stress views of both shoulders with a 10 lb weight in the

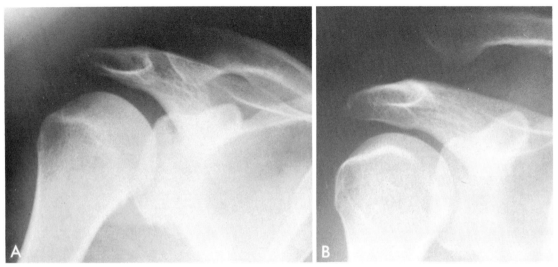

**Figure 3–12.** Acromioclavicular separation is demonstrated on the erect film *(B)* but is not seen in the supine radiograph *(A)*.

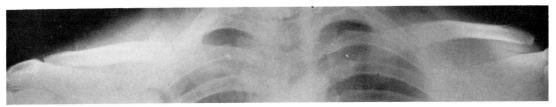

**Figure 3–13.** A Type II acromioclavicular separation is indicated by minimal elevation of the clavicle and/or widening of the acromioclavicular joint as noted on the left.

hands show no widening of the coracoclavicular space. This type of injury may be treated by closed or open methods, including arthroplasty or excision of the distal 2 cm of the clavicle.[26]

A Type III injury shows widening of the acromioclavicular joint and elevation of the distal clavicle completely above the acromion process due to disruption of the acromioclavicular and coracoclavicular ligaments. Stress views show a marked difference in the coracoclavicular distance between the two sides (Fig. 3–14). This type of injury is treated operatively by acromioclavicular or coracoclavicular repair or by excision of the distal 2 cm of the clavicle. Acromioclavicular repair includes fixation of the acromioclavicular joint by Steinmann pins, the lateral portion of the pin being bent to prevent migration. Coracoclavicular repair includes fixation between the clavicle and the coracoid process by screws or wires (Fig. 3–15).[25, 27]

Complications of these operative techniques that may be observed radiographically include acromioclavicular joint arthritis, soft tissue calcification, bone resorption around the metal, metal failure, inadequate bony purchase of the metallic fixation, fracture of the bone through the implant holes, and migration of pins and wires.[28–30]

### Dislocation of the Sternoclavicular Joint

Dislocation of the sternoclavicular joint is rare, more commonly occurring anteriorly than posteriorly, and it is difficult to demonstrate radiographically. Rockwood proposes an anteroposterior radiographic projection with the tube tilted 40° toward the head and centered to the manubrium (Fig. 3–16). Tube-patient distance is 45 inches in children and 60 inches in adults. Anterior dislocation of the sternoclavicular joint is manifested by superior displacement of the clavicular head and posterior dislocation by inferior displacement of the clavicular head (Fig. 3–16B). Sternoclavicular dislocation may be treated by pin or Kirschner wire

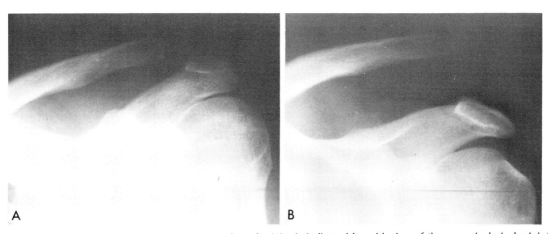

A                                        B

**Figure 3–14.** A Type III injury of the acromioclavicular joint is indicated by widening of the acromioclavicular joint and elevation of the distal clavicle above the acromion process as well as an increased coracoclavicular distance. The stress view *(B)* demonstrates what might have been called a Type II injury on the nonstress view *(A)* to be a Type III injury.

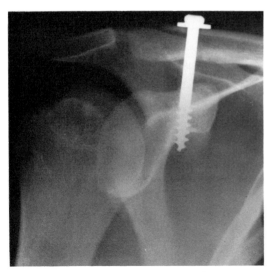

**Figure 3–15.** Screw fixation indicates that a coracoclavicular repair has been performed.

fixation from the clavicle into the manubrium; however, resection of the medial aspect of the clavicle may be performed for recurrent or unreduced dislocation.[31]

## DISORDERS OF THE HUMERUS

### Glenohumeral Joint Disease

Although total joint arthroplasty or humeral head replacement has not been ideal in restoring full range of motion and function to the glenohumeral joint affected by rheumatoid arthritis, it has been very effective in the relief of pain (Fig. 3–17).[32] Cephalad subluxation of the humeral head on the radiograph indicates rupture of the rotator cuff and instability. A total joint arthroplasty will contribute greater stability in these cases than humeral head replacement alone.[33]

### Fractures of the Proximal Humerus

Fractures of the proximal humerus occur more commonly in the elderly patient and more recently have been classified by the orthopedic surgeon according to segmental displacement or angulation in an effort to determine treatment required. This classification, known as the Four-Segment Classification, is based on dividing the proximal humerus into four anatomic segments: (1) the greater tuberosity segment, (2) the lesser tuberosity segment, (3) the articular or anatomic neck segment, and (4) the shaft or surgical neck segment (Fig. 3–18).[6]

Displacement of a segment greater than 1 cm or angulation of a segment greater than 45 degrees constitutes a *displaced fracture*. Displacement less than 1 cm constitutes minimum displacement. According to this

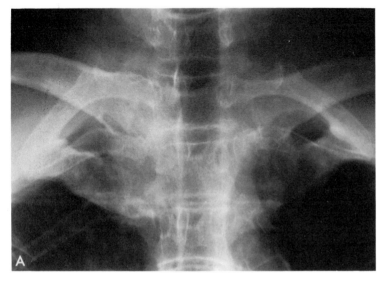

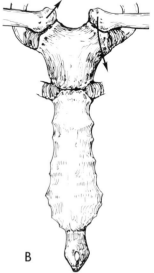

B

**Figure 3–16.** *A*, An anteroposterior view with the tube angled 40 degrees cephalad and centered to the manubrium will demonstrate sternoclavicular dislocation when present. The sternoclavicular joints are normally aligned in this case. *B*, Diagram of anterior and posterior sternoclavicular dislocation. Displacement of the right clavicular head superiorly would indicate anterior dislocation; of the left clavicular head inferiorly, posterior dislocation.

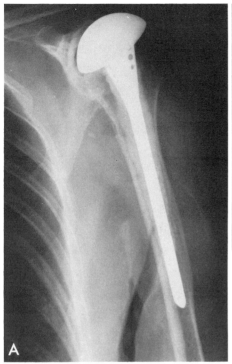

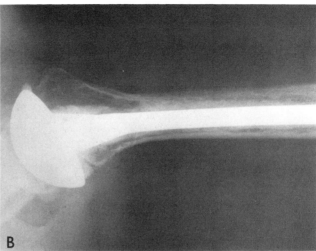

**Figure 3–17.** Total joint arthroplasty of the shoulder for rheumatoid arthritis.

classification, a *one-part fracture* consists of minimal displacement, a *two-part fracture* consists of displacement of one segment, a *three-part fracture,* displacement of two segments, and a *four-part fracture* consists of displacement of all four segments.[6]

*Radiographic evaluation* of fractures of the shoulder requires an anteroposterior and an axillary or scapulotangential lateral view. The axillary view demonstrates glenoid and coracoid process fractures, which may be difficult to see on other views (Fig. 3–19). The scapulotangential lateral view is effec-

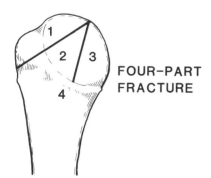

FOUR–PART
FRACTURE

**Figure 3–18.** Four-segment classification of fractures of the proximal humerus. (1) Greater tuberosity segment, (2) Lesser tuberosity segment, (3) Articular or anatomic neck segment, and (4) Shaft or surgical neck segment.

tive when the patient is in severe pain, precluding any movement of the shoulder.[7]

Treatment based on the Four-Segment Classification consists of passive exercises for minimally displaced fractures, closed reduction for two-part fractures, open reduction for three-part fractures, and a humeral head prosthesis for four-part fractures (Table 3–1).

**Complications of Fractures of the Proximal Humerus.** Fractures of the proximal humerus usually unite unless markedly displaced or distracted. Excessive distraction, as may occur from treatment by a hanging cast, may lead to nonunion.[8–10]

### Fractures of the Distal Humerus

Fractures of the distal humerus may be classified anatomically as supracondylar, transcondylar (dicondylar), intercondylar (T or Y), condylar, epicondylar, or articular surface only (Fig. 3–20).

**Intercondylar Fractures.** Intercondylar fractures have been further classified on the basis of radiographic appearance into four types to provide a guide for the orthopedic surgeon to management and prognosis (Fig.

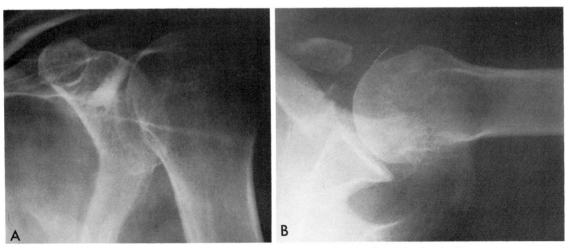

**Figure 3–19.** Coracoid process fracture was seen only on axillary lateral projection.

**Table 3–1.** FOUR-SEGMENT CLASSIFICATION OF PROXIMAL HUMERAL
FRACTURES AND TREATMENT

| Classification | X-ray Appearance | Treatment |
| --- | --- | --- |
| One-part fracture | Minimal displacement (less than 1 cm) | Passive exercises |
| Two-part fracture | Displacement (greater than 1 cm) of one segment | Closed reduction |
| Three-part fracture | Displacement (greater than 1 cm) of two segments | Open reduction and internal fixation |
| Four-part fracture | Displacement (greater than 1 cm) of all four segments | Humeral head prosthesis |

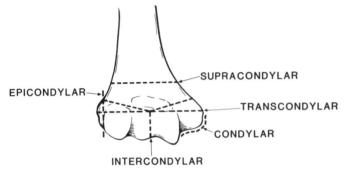

**Figure 3–20.** Anatomic classification of distal humerus fractures.

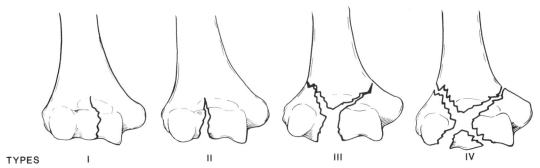

**Figure 3–21.** Classification of intercondylar fractures.

3–21). Type I is an undisplaced fracture between the capitellum and trochlea. A Type II fracture indicates a separation of the capitellum and trochlea without appreciable rotation of the fragments in the frontal plane. In Type III fractures there is separation of the fragments with rotary deformity. A Type IV fracture has severe comminution of the articular surface with wide separation of the humeral condyles. Treatment of distal humeral fractures may be nonoperative or operative, depending upon the patient and the type of injury. Operative treatment of intercondylar fractures includes pins in plaster, open reduction and internal fixation, arthroplasty, and prosthetic (distal humerus) replacement (Fig. 3–22).[35–38]

## Fractures of the Humeral Condyles

Fractures of the humeral condyles (medial or lateral) have also been classified according to extent of fracture through the lateral

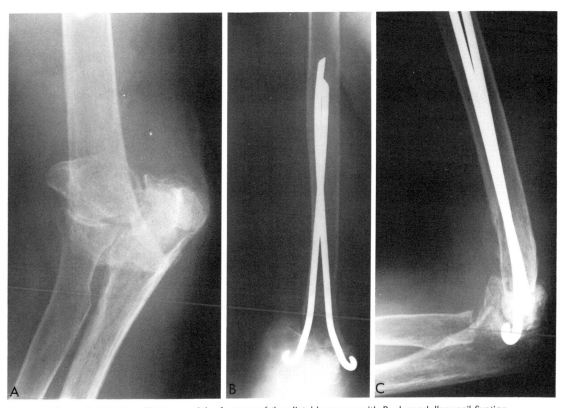

**Figure 3–22.** Type III intercondylar fracture of the distal humerus with Rush medullary nail fixation.

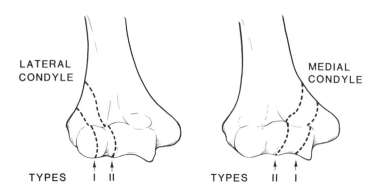

**Figure 3–23.** Classification of humeral condyle fractures.

trochlear ridge (Fig. 3–23). This classification aids in selection of treatment and determination of potential for medial-lateral instability of the elbow. The Type I fracture spares the lateral trochlear ridge, whereas the Type II fracture extends through the lateral trochlear ridge, allowing medial-lateral dislocation between the humerus and the radius and ulna. Type I fractures may or may not require operative treatment, while Type II fractures do require open reduction and internal fixation. Complications of condylar fractures include alignment abnormalities such as cubitus valgus and cubitus varus, as well as post-traumatic arthritis.[39]

## DISORDERS OF THE ELBOW

### Dislocations of the Elbow

Dislocations of the elbow are most commonly posterior or posterolateral. Adequate reduction is indicated by alignment of the radial head with the humeral condyles in the lateral projection, so that a line drawn through the central axis of the radius intersects the articular surface of the humeral condyles (Fig. 3–24).[40–43]

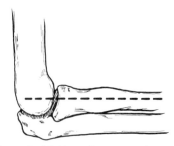

**Figure 3–24.** Normal anatomic alignment of elbow on lateral view.

### Fractures of the Olecranon Process

Fractures of the olecranon process may be undisplaced or displaced, 2 mm or more of separation constituting displacement.[44] Displaced fractures resulting from pull of the triceps tendon usually require open reduction with internal fixation, such as intramedullary fixation (wood screws, threaded Steinmann pins, Rush rods), bicortical screw fixation (cortical screw passes through posterior cortex of olecranon process and anterior cortex of coronoid process) (Figs. 3–25 and 3–26), tension band wiring (figure-of-eight wire passes around insertion of triceps tendon, goes distally beyond fracture site and through the olecranon process) (Fig. 3–27), and excision of the proximal fragments. When excision is performed, the triceps tendon is reattached to the distal fragment.[45–48] Olecranon fractures may also be complicated by nonunion or degenerative arthritis of the elbow (Fig. 3–28).

### Fractures of the Radial Head

Fractures of the head of the radius have been classified into three types, depending upon the amount of displacement and the extent of the fracture (Fig. 3–29). Type I fractures are undisplaced. Problems classified as Type II are marginal fractures with displacement (including impaction, depression, and angulation). Type III fractures are comminuted, involving the entire head.[49] A fracture of the radial head may not be visualized initially, but a positive fat pad sign should suggest this diagnosis and follow-up films should be obtained (Fig. 3–30). Fracture fragments observed proximal to the ra-

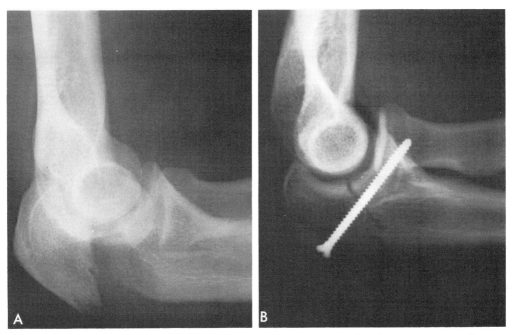

**Figure 3–25.** Bicortical screw fixation of fracture of olecranon process. Note that the screw engages the posterior cortex of the olecranon process and the anterior cortex of the coronoid process.

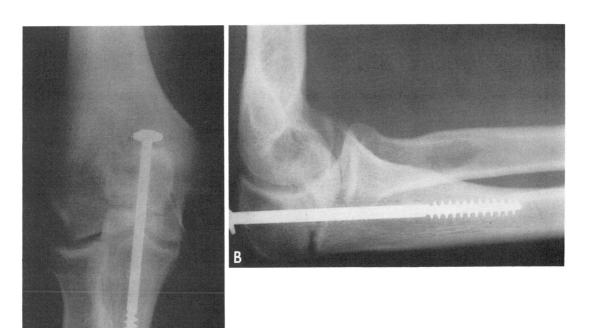

**Figure 3–26.** *A* and *B,* Internal fixation of a fracture of the olecranon process of the ulna. Screw fixation with subsequent nonunion.

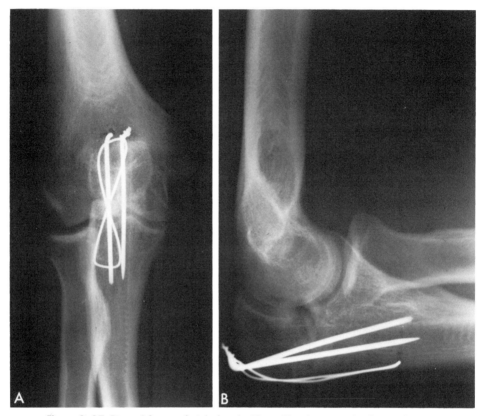

**Figure 3–27.** Pin and figure-of-eight band wiring with subsequent healing and union.

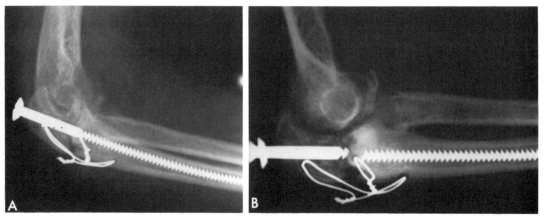

**Figure 3–28.** Screw fixation of an olecranon fracture with subsequent fracture of the screw and nonunion.

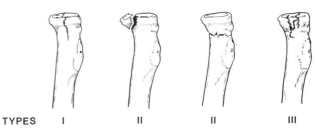

**Figure 3–29.** Classification of fractures of the head of the radius (see text).

TYPES    I        II        II        III

dial head on the lateral view represent a fracture of the capitellum, even though the radial head may be fractured.[50] Treatment of radial head fractures is nonoperative for Type I injuries. Excision of the radial head for significant angulation, depression, or extent is best for Type II and Type III injuries.[51]

Subluxation of the distal radioulnar joint may occur following radial head excision or nonoperative management of radial head fractures and may or may not be symptomatic.[52]

Arthritic changes in the elbow and distal forearm are commonly observed in rheumatoid and post-traumatic arthritis. Excision of the radial head is performed in cases of severe rheumatoid arthritis to provide pain relief and increased range of motion. A Silastic radial head prosthesis may be implanted to maintain alignment (Fig. 3–31). Persistent limitation of rotational movement of the forearm due to involvement of the distal radioulnar joint may be effectively relieved by resection of the distal 2 to 3 cm of the ulna (Darrach procedure). Excessive resection of the distal ulna, however, may

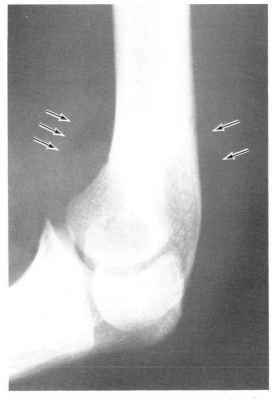

**Figure 3–30.** Positive fat pad sign (arrows) in the absence of a radiographically demonstrable fracture of the radial head necessitates an interval examination in seven to ten days to exclude a subtle fracture if symptoms persist.

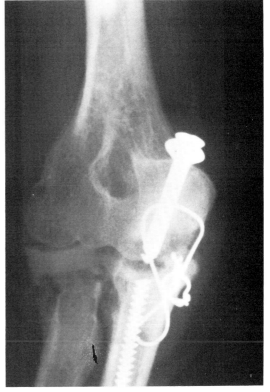

**Figure 3–31.** A silastic radial head prosthesis is implanted to maintain alignment following excision of the radial head.

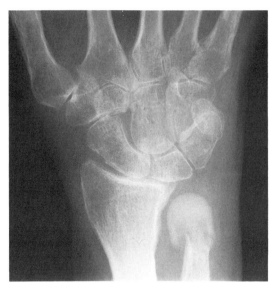

**Figure 3–32.** Darrach procedure consists of resection of the distal 2 to 3 cm of the ulna to increase the range of motion of the wrist. Ulnar head implant is present to prevent carpal shift and instability.

result in instability and ulnar shift of the carpal bones. For this reason, a concomitant ulnar head implant is performed to maintain the physiologic length of the ulna and to prevent ulnar carpal shift and instability (Fig. 3–32).

## Arthritis of the Elbow

Total joint arthroplasty of the elbow is presently not as advanced as that of the hip and knee and is subject to various complications such as loosening and fracture. Painful loosening following a hinge type of prosthesis may occur at the cement-bone interface of the humeral component (Fig. 3–33).[54]

## Tennis Elbow

Tennis elbow is a syndrome characterized by pain over the lateral epicondyle of the humerus usually in individuals subjected to frequent rotary motion of the forearm. The cause is unknown and the radiographs are negative. Treatment may be conservative or surgical.[66, 67]

## Osteochondritis Dissecans of the Elbow

Osteochondritis dissecans of the elbow more commonly occurs in the capitellum and is radiographically recognized as an area of decreased density, punched-out defect, or irregular sclerosis on the articular surface.

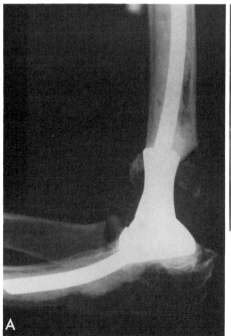
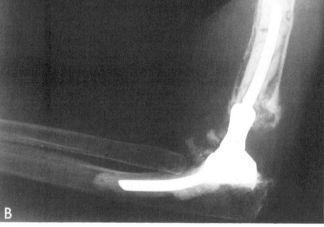

**Figure 3–33.** Loosening of a hinge-type total elbow prosthesis. *A,* Preloosening. *B,* Postloosening; note fractures in methacrylate and increased lucency between methacrylate and bone.

Surgery is indicated when locking occurs owing to loose bodies or early degenerative arthritis.[68]

## DISORDERS OF THE FOREARM

### Fractures of the Forearm

Fractures of the forearm most commonly involve both the radius and ulna, and axial and rotational alignment must be restored if full and adequate range of motion is to result. At times in children, only one of the paired bones may fracture with subsequent dissipation of the stress, resulting in acute plastic bowing of the opposite bone (Fig. 3–34). If this bowing is not reduced, pronation and supination may be restricted.[57, 58] In order to reduce forearm fractures adequately and to maintain the reduction and alignment, open reduction and internal fixation with intramedullary nails or compression plate and screws are usually required for

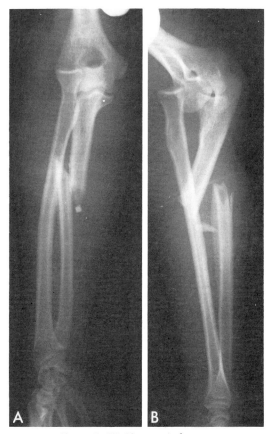

**Figure 3–35.** Monteggia fracture.

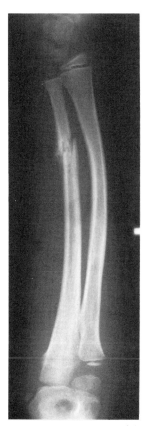

**Figure 3–34.** Acute plastic bowing of the radius associated with a fracture of the distal ulna.

displaced diaphyseal fractures in the adult.[59–62]

Two specific fracture dislocations of the forearm that exemplify the rule that dissipation of stress occurs either by fracture of both paired bones or fractures of one paired bone and dislocation of the other are the Monteggia and Galeazzi fractures.

The Monteggia fracture is a usually anteriorly angulated fracture of the proximal third of the ulna in association with an anterior dislocation of the radial head (Fig. 3–35). Variations that may occur and can be considered as Monteggia lesions include a posteriorly angulated fracture of the shaft of the ulna associated with a posterior dislocation of the radial head, a fracture of the ulnar metaphysis in association with lateral or anterolateral dislocation of the radial head, or fractures of the proximal third of the radius and ulna at the same level associated with anterior dislocation of the radial head.[63, 64]

The Galeazzi fracture consists of a usually dorsally angulated fracture of the junction

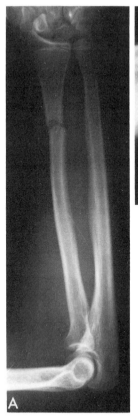
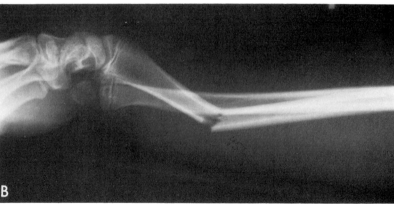

**Figure 3–36.** Galeazzi fracture.

of the middle and distal thirds of the radius in association with dislocation of the radioulnar joint (Fig. 3–36).

Complications of forearm fractures include nonunion, malunion, infection, compartment syndrome (anterior or posterior) similar to that in the leg, and synostosis between the radius and ulna.[65]

## References

1. Kotzen LM: Roentgen diagnosis of rotator cuff tear. AJR 112:507–511, 1971
2. Killoran PJ, Marcove RC, Freiberger RH: Shoulder arthrography. AJR 103:658–668, 1968
3. Goldman AB, Ghelman G: The double-contrast shoulder arthrogram. Radiology 127:655–663, 1978
4. Freiberger RH, Kaye JJ: Arthrography. Appleton-Century-Crofts, New York, 1979, p. 140
5. Gilula LA, Schoenecker PL, Murphy WA: Shoulder arthrography as a treatment modality. AJR 131:1047–1048, 1978
6. Neer CS II: Displacement proximal humeral fractures. Part I. Classification and evaluation. J Bone Joint Surg 52A:1077–1089, 1970
7. Rubin SA, Gray RL, Green WR: Scapular Y-diagnostic aid in shoulder trauma. Radiology 110:725–726, 1974
8. Hundley JM, Stewart MJ: Fractures of the humerus: a comparative study in methods of treatment. J Bone Joint Surg 37A:681–692, 1955
9. Whitson TB: Fractures of the surgical neck of the humerus—a study in reduction. J Bone Joint Surg 36B:423–427, 1954
10. Neer CS II: Prosthetic replacement of the humeral head—indications and operative technique. Surg Clin N Am 43:1581–1597, 1963
11. Turek SL: Orthopaedics: Principles and Their Application. 3rd ed. J. B. Lippincott Co., Philadelphia, 1977, pp. 842–850
12. Hill HA, Sachs MD: The grooved defect of the humeral head. A frequently unrecognized complication of dislocation of the shoulder joint. Radiology 35:690–700, 1940
13. Hall RH, Isaac F, Booth DR: Dislocation of the shoulder with special reference to accompanying small fractures. J Bone Joint Surg 41A:489–494, 1959
14. Osmond-Clarke H: Habitual dislocation of the shoulder. The Putti-Platt operation. J Bone Joint Surg 30B:19–25, 1948
15. Bankart ASB: Recurrent or habitual dislocation of the shoulder joint. Br Med J 2:1132–1133, 1923
16. Magnuson PB: Treatment of recurrent dislocation of the shoulder. Surg Clin N Am 25:14–20, 1945
17. Magnuson PB, Stack JK: Recurrent dislocation of the shoulder. JAMA 123:898–892, 1943
18. Lombardo SJ, Kerlan RK, Jobe FW, Carter VS, Blazina ME, Shields CL: The modified Bristow procedure for recurrent dislocation of the shoulder. J Bone Joint Surg 58A:256–261, 1976
19. Neer CS II: Fracture of the distal clavicle with detachment of the coracoclavicular ligaments in adults. J Trauma 3:99–110, 1968

20. Neer CS II: Fractures of the distal third of the clavicle. Clin Orthop 58:43–50, 1968

21. Seymour EQ: Osteolysis of the clavicular tip associated with repeated minor trauma to the shoulder. Radiology 123:56, 1977

22. Halaby FA, DiSalvo EL: Osteolysis: a complication of trauma. Report of 2 cases. AJR 94:591–594, 1965

23. Madsen B: Osteolysis of the acromial end of the clavicle following trauma. Br J Radiol 36:822–826, 1963

24. Bosworth BM: Complete acromioclavicular dislocation. New Engl J Med 241:221–225, 1949

25. Bearden JM, Hughston JC, Whatley GS: Acromioclavicular dislocation: method of treatment. J Sports Med 1:5–17, 1973

26. Mumford EB: Acromioclavicular dislocation. J Bone Joint Surg 23:799–802, 1941

27. Allredge RH: Surgical treatment of acromioclavicular dislocations. J Bone Joint Surg 47A:1278, 1965

28. Rockwood CA: Dislocations about the shoulder. In Rockwood CA, Green DP: Fractures. Vol. 1. JB Lippincott Co., Philadelphia, 1975, pp. 721–756

29. Mazet RJ: Migration of a Kirschner wire from the shoulder region into the lung. Report of 2 cases. J Bone Joint Surg 25A:477–483, 1943

30. Norrell H, Llewellyn RD: Migration of a threaded Steinmann pin from an acromioclavicular joint into the spinal canal. A case report. J Bone Joint Surg 47A:1024–1026, 1965

31. Rockwood CA: Dislocations about the shoulder. In Rockwood CA, Green DP: Fractures. Vol. 1. JB Lippincott Co., Philadelphia, 1975, p. 769

32. Marmor L: Arthritis Surgery. Lea & Febiger, Philadelphia, 1976

33. Marmor L: Hemiarthroplasty for the rheumatoid shoulder joint. Clin Orthop 122:201–203, 1977

34. Roper, BA: Complications of arthroplasty and total joint replacement in the shoulder. In Epps CH Jr: Complications in Orthopaedic Surgery. JB Lippincott Co., Philadelphia, 1978, pp. 853–857

35. Riseborough EJ, Radin EL: Intercondylar T-fractures of the humerus in the adult. A comparison of operative and non-operative treatment in twenty-nine cases. J Bone Joint Surg 51A:130–141, 1969

36. Miller WA: Comminuted fractures of the distal end of the humerus in the adult. J Bone Joint Surg 46A:644–657, 1964

37. Watson-Jones R: Fractures and Joint Injuries. 3rd ed. Vol. 2. Williams and Wilkins, Baltimore, 1946

38. Barr JS, Erton RG: Elbow reconstruction with a new prosthesis to replace the distal end of the humerus. J Bone Joint Surg 47A:1408–1413, 1965

39. Milch H: Fracture and fracture dislocations of the humeral condyles. J Trauma 4:592–607, 1964

40. Kini MG: Dislocation of the elbow and its complications. J Bone Joint Surg 22:107–117, 1940

41. Linscheid RL, Wheeler DK: Elbow dislocation. JAMA 194:1171–1176, 1965

42. Conn J, Wade PA: Injuries of the elbow—a ten year review. J Trauma 1:248–268, 1961

43. Vesley DG: Isolated traumatic dislocations of the radial head in children. Clin Orthop, 50:31–36, 1967

44. Eriksson E, Sahlen O, Sandohl U: Late results of conservative and surgical treatment of fracture of the olecranon. Acta Chir Scand 113:153–166, 1957

45. Harmon PH: Treatment of fractures of the olecranon by fixation with stainless steel screws. J Bone Joint Surg 27:328–329, 1945

46. Taylor TKF, Scham SM: A posteromedial approach to the proximal end of the ulna for the internal fixation of olecranon fracture. J Trauma 9:594–602, 1969

47. Müller ME, Allgöner M, Willenegger H: Manual of Internal Fixation. Springer-Verlag, New York, 1970

48. Adler S, Fay GF, MacAusland WR Jr: Treatment of olecranon fractures. Indication for excision of the olecranon fragment and repair of the triceps tendon. J Trauma 2:597–602, 1962

49. Mason ML: Some observations on fractures of the head and the radius with a review of one hundred cases. Br J Surg 42:123–132, 1954

50. Milch H: Unusual fractures of the capitulum humeri and the capitulum radii. J Bone Joint Surg 13:882, 1931.

51. Epright RH, Wilkins FE: Fractures and dislocations of the elbow. In Rockwood CA, Green DP: Fractures. Vol. 1. JB Lippincott Co., Philadelphia, 1975, pp. 487–584

52. Radin EL, Riseborough EJ: A review of eighty-eight cases and analysis of the indications for excision of the radial head and non-operative treatment. J Bone Joint Surg 48A:1055–1064, 1966

53. Swanson AB, Herndon JH, Swanson, G: Complications of arthroplasty and joint replacement at the wrist. In Epps CH Jr: Complications in Orthopaedic Surgery. JB Lippincott Co., Philadelphia, 1978, pp. 873–903

54. Bryan RS: Total joint replacement of the elbow joint. Arch Surg 112:1092–1093, 1977

55. Turek SL: Orthopaedics: Principles and Their Application. 3rd ed. JB Lippincott Co., Philadelphia, 1977, p. 880

56. Taylor AR, Mukerjea SK, Rana NA: Excision of the head of the radius in rheumatoid arthritis. J Bone Joint Surg 58B:485, 1976

57. Borden S IV: Roentgen recognition of acute plastic bowing of the forearm in children. AJR 125:524–530, 1975

58. Crowe JE, Swischuk LE: Acute bowing fractures of the forearm in children: a frequently missed injury. AJR 128:981–984, 1977

59. Dodge HS, Cody GW: Treatment of fractures of the radius and ulna with compression plates: a retrospective study of one-hundred eight patients. J Bone Joint Surg 54A:1167–1176, 1972

60. Smith JEM: Internal fixation in the treatment of fractures of the shaft of the radius and ulna in adults. J Bone Joint Surg 41B:122–131, 1959

61. Sage FP: Medullary fixation of fractures of the forearm. A study of the medullary canal of the radius and a report of fifty fractures of the radius treated with a prebent triangular nail. J Bone Joint Surg 41A:1489–1516, 1959

62. Naiman PT, Schein AJ, Seiffert RS: Use of ASIF compression plates in selected shaft fractures of the upper extremity. Clin Orthop 71:208–217, 1970

63. Bado JL: The Monteggia lesion. Clin Orthop 50:71–76, 1967

64. Boyd HB, Boals JO: The Monteggia lesion. A review of 159 cases. Clin Orthop 66:94–100, 1969

65. Anderson LD, Sisk TD, Park WI, Tooms RE: Compression plate fixation in acute diaphyseal fractures of the radius and ulna. J Bone Joint Surg 54A:1332–1333, 1972

66. Bosworth DM: The role of the orbicular ligament in tennis elbow. J Bone Joint Surg 37A:527, 1955

67. Spencer GE Jr, Herndon CH: Surgical treatment of epicondylitis. J Bone Joint Surg 35A:421, 1953

68. Roberts R, Hughes R: Osteochondritis dessicans of the elbow joint. J Bone Joint Surg 32B:348, 1950

# 4

# THE HAND AND WRIST

Orthopedic radiographic evaluation of the hand and wrist is most commonly performed for trauma and nonrheumatoid and rheumatoid diseases. Whereas conventional radiography is most often utilized in this evaluation, magnification has provided better delineation of the early arthritic changes and subtle fractures[1, 2] (Fig. 4–1).

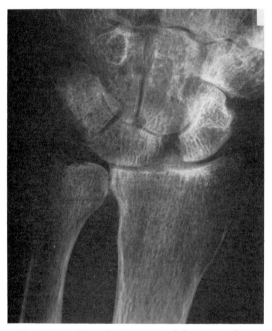

**Figure 4–1.** Magnification view of the wrist utilizing a microfocal spot tube demonstrates early erosive changes in the carpal bones in a patient with rheumatoid arthritis. Note the excellent trabecular detail. (Courtesy of Dr. Donald Resnick, San Diego, California.)

## TRAUMA

### Fractures in the Radius and Ulna

A comminuted fracture of the distal radial metaphysis with dorsal displacement of the distal fragment (Colles fracture) is a common injury to the wrist. There is frequently an associated fracture through the ulnar styloid and loss of the normal palmar angulation (5 to 15 degrees) of the distal radius (Fig. 4–2).

Closed reduction is the usual method of treatment, and postreduction films should demonstrate correction of the dorsal displacement and restoration of the distal radial angulation to at least the neutral position (Fig. 4–3). Interval postreduction films are necessary to check the position of the fracture fragments when there is extensive comminution because movement of the fragments is enhanced. Nonunion is uncommon, while malunion occurs frequently. Fracture of the dorsal lip of the distal radial articular surface (Barton fracture) is best delineated on the lateral view. The fracture fragment is displaced proximally and dorsally (Fig. 4–4). Like the Colles fracture, it is treated by closed reduction.[6]

A fracture through the radial styloid (Hutchinson fracture) may also occur and is treated by closed reduction. Fracture of the distal radial metaphysis with anterior displacement and accentuated palmar angulation of the distal fracture fragment, best seen on the lateral projection, constitutes the Smith or reverse Colles fracture and is usually treated by closed reduction[6] (Fig. 4–4).

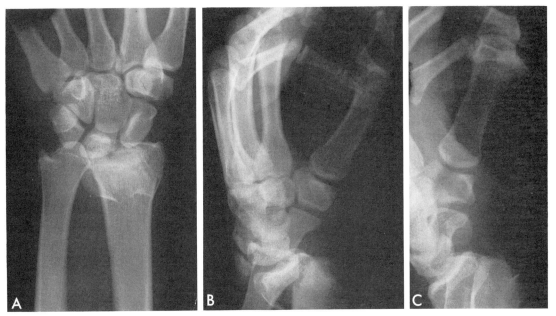

**Figure 4–2.** *A* to *C,* The Colles fracture is a fracture complex consisting of a comminuted fracture of the distal radius with dorsal displacement of the distal fracture fragments, volar angulation, and commonly a fracture of the ulnar styloid.

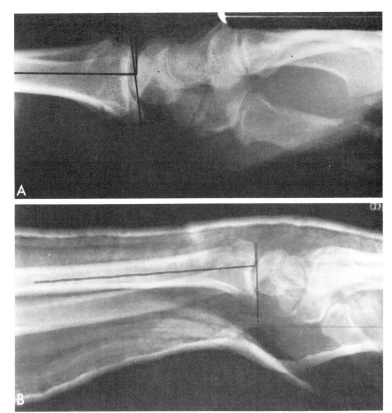

**Figure 4–3.** *A* and *B,* Postreduction films demonstrate restoration of distal radial articular surface angulation to the neutral position from an 8° dorsal tilt. Normally, the articular surface has a palmar tilt.

## FRACTURES

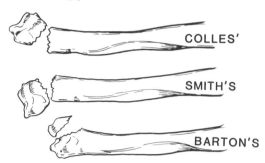

**Figure 4–4.** Diagrammatic representation of Colles, Smith, and Barton fractures of the distal radius seen in lateral projection.

Ulnar styloid fractures may occur singly or in combination with other fractures and are significant if associated with damage to the triangular cartilage.[7, 8]

### Fractures of the Wrist

Fracture of the navicular bone most commonly occurs through the waist or middle third of the navicular. A special navicular view, distorting and elongating the navicular bone, or magnification will optimally delineate subtle or hairline fractures obscured on conventional views[9] (Fig. 4–5). If, however, original films are negative for a fracture and tenderness persists in the region of the anatomic snuff box, the patient is treated as if a fracture were present and repeat films at two- and four-week intervals are recommended. Since the blood supply of the navicular enters the distal aspect of the bone, avascular necrosis of the proximal fragment can occur with motion at the fracture site. Radiographic evidence of healing is usually observed by the sixth week.[10, 11, 12, 13]

Complications of navicular fractures include delayed union, nonunion, and avascular necrosis (Fig. 4–6). Delayed union is recognized radiographically by resorption along the fracture margins as well as by cystic and sclerotic changes. Treatment may be closed, requiring immobilization for one year or more for union to occur, or open, requiring internal fixation (Kirschner wires, corticocancellous bone screws) if displacement persists, or bone grafting, or both.[10, 14] When Kirschner wires are used, the protruding external portion is bent at right angles to prevent migration of the wires. Nonunion

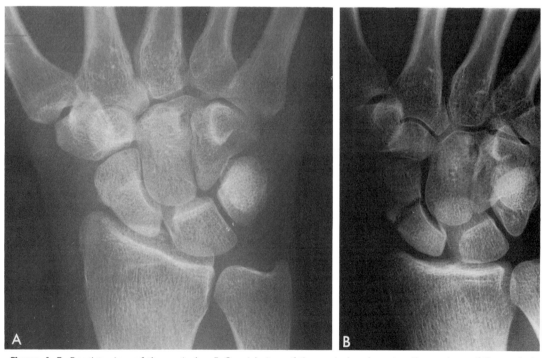

**Figure 4–5.** Routine view of the navicular. *B,* Special view of the navicular elongates the contour of the navicular bone, allowing fractures to be better delineated.

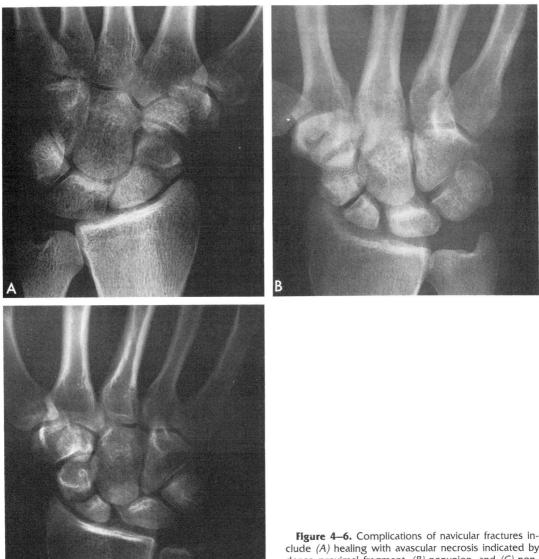

**Figure 4–6.** Complications of navicular fractures include (A) healing with avascular necrosis indicated by dense proximal fragment, (B) nonunion, and (C) nonunion with avascular necrosis.

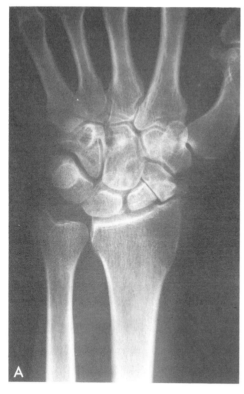

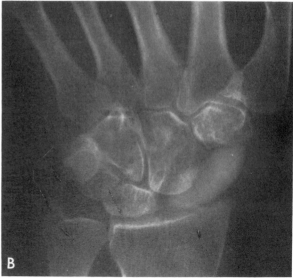

**Figure 4–7.** Navicular implant. Nonunion of navicular fracture and post-traumatic arthritis *(A)*, treated by a silicone navicular implant *(B)*.

is treated by bone grafting if the proximal fracture fragment is viable or necrotic provided arthritis is not present. If arthritis is already present, an arthrodesis is performed.[12, 15] A navicular implant (Fig. 4–7) may also be used in the treatment of nonunion, markedly comminuted acute fractures, pseudarthrosis, and failure of previous surgery.[16]

**Carpal Dislocation-Dissociation.** When a carpal fracture is observed, an associated dislocation or dissociation should also be suspected. These include a transscaphoid perilunate dislocation, perilunate dislocation, lunate dislocation, and rotary subluxation of the scaphoid. The transscaphoid perilunate dislocation is the most common carpal dislocation, characterized by a fracture of the waist of the navicular and dorsal dislocation of the carpal bones except for the lunate, which remains in normal position to the distal radius (Fig. 4–8 A and B). The perilunate dislocation is characterized by dorsal dislocation of the carpal bones with normal relationship between the lunate and distal radius maintained (Fig. 4–8 C and D), whereas the lunate dislocation is char-

acterized by volar dislocation of the lunate with normal relationship maintained between the other carpal bones and the distal radius (Fig. 4–8 E and F). Both perilunate and lunate dislocations may be associated with rotary subluxation of the navicular, which is characterized by abnormal widening of the distance between the navicular and lunate and is important because of its complication by post-traumatic arthritis (Fig. 4–8 G).

Avascular necrosis of the lunate (Kienböck's disease), whether idiopathic or resulting from trauma, may also be treated by a Silastic implant that functions as a spacer maintaining carpal bone relationships (Fig. 4–9).[18]

## Fractures of the Hand

Fractures of the metacarpals are adequately evaluated by anteroposterior and oblique projections, whereas phalangeal fractures require anteroposterior, lateral, and oblique views.

Most metacarpal and phalangeal fractures

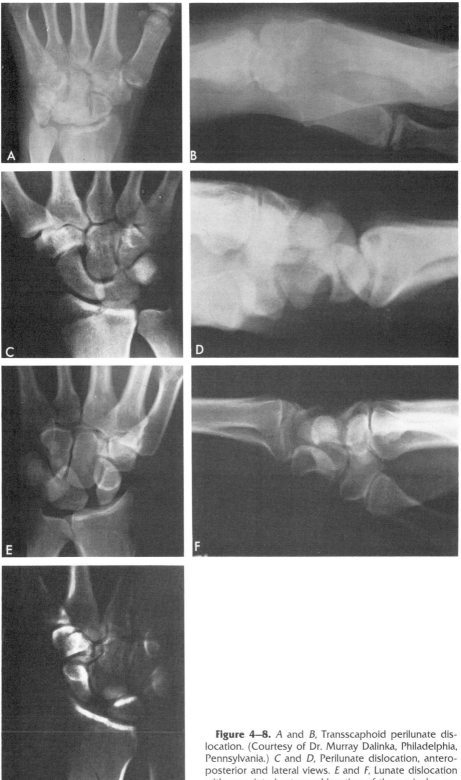

**Figure 4–8.** *A* and *B*, Transscaphoid perilunate dislocation. (Courtesy of Dr. Murray Dalinka, Philadelphia, Pennsylvania.) *C* and *D*, Perilunate dislocation, anteroposterior and lateral views. *E* and *F*, Lunate dislocation with associated rotary subluxation of the navicular, anteroposterior *(E)* and lateral *(F)* views. *G*, Rotary subluxation of the scaphoid.

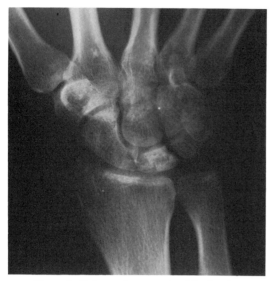

**Figure 4–9.** Avascular necrosis of the lunate.

most commonly requires internal fixation with Kirschner wires (Fig. 4–10 A). A comminuted Bennett fracture, or Rolando fracture, may be treated by open reduction if the comminuted fragments are large, and by closed reduction if the fragments are small (Fig. 4–10 B). Extra-articular fractures of the first metacarpal are most commonly treated by closed reduction, while transverse fractures of the second through fifth metacarpal shafts usually require Kirschner wire fixation because of dorsal angulation owing to interosseous muscle pull (Fig. 4–11).

Metacarpal head fractures are treated by closed reduction, but metacarpal neck fractures may be sufficently unstable to require open reduction and internal fixation. Phalangeal fractures may involve the distal, middle, or proximal phalanges. Longitudinal, transverse, or comminuted fractures are frequently observed in the distal phalanx. A flexion deformity (mallet finger) of the distal interphalangeal joint may occur as a result of disruption of the extensor tendon to the distal phalanx or after a fracture involving one third or more of the dorsal articular surface of the distal phalanx. It is treated by splinting (Fig. 4–12).

are stable and are therefore treated by closed reduction. Some require Kirschner wire or pin fixation, however, because of instability. The Bennett fracture, involving the base of the first metacarpal and extending into the carpometacarpal joint, is associated with a radial dislocation of the metacarpal and

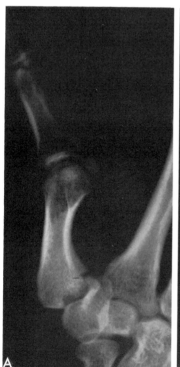

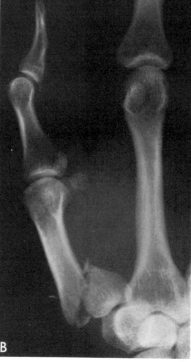

**Figure 4–10.** *A*, Bennett fracture. *B*, Rolando fracture.

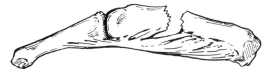

**Figure 4–11.** Interosseous muscle pull exerts a volar force, resulting in dorsal angulation of the metacarpal and necessitating wire fixation.

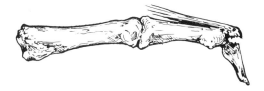

**Figure 4–12.** Mallet finger deformity.

Fractures of the middle and proximal phalanges are classified as extra-articular or intra-articular (Fig. 4–13). Those fractures most likely to be unstable, and therefore requiring internal fixation with Kirschner wires, are (1) long oblique extra-articular fractures of the proximal phalanx, (2) displaced fractures of one or both condyles of the proximal or middle phalanx, (3) large displaced intra-articular marginal fractures of the base of the proximal phalanx, or (4) displaced avulsion fractures with associated boutonnière deformity.[20, 21]

Volar plate fractures are usually best seen on the lateral view. They result from avulsion of the insertion of the volar capsule, usually in a hyperextension injury. Open reduction and internal fixation may be re-

quired if the fracture fragment is large (Fig. 4–14).[22]

Dislocations and ligamentous injuries of the metacarpal, phalangeal, and interphalangeal joints are commonly observed in association with fractures. Stress views are helpful in determining ligamentous injuries; however, comparison with the opposite finger should be made. Posterior dislocation is most commonly observed, and closed reduction is the most common method of treatment. Metacarpophalangeal dislocations characterized by widening of the joint space and interposition of the sesamoid bone between the metacarpal and the proximal phalanx indicate displacement of the volar plate within the joint and require operative reduction.[23, 24]

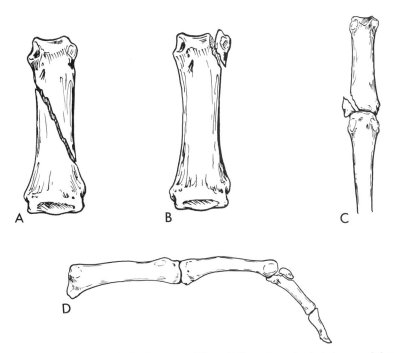

**Figure 4–13.** Extra-articular and intra-articular fractures of the middle and proximal phalanges. *A,* Long oblique extra-articular fracture of the proximal phalanx. *B,* A displaced fracture of one or both condyles of the proximal or middle phalanx. *C,* Large displaced intra-articular marginal fractures of the base of the proximal phalanx. *D,* A displaced avulsion fracture with associated boutonniere deformity.

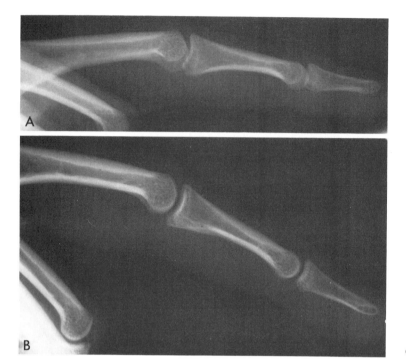

**Figure 4–14.** Volar plate fracture. Oblique *(A)* and lateral *(B)* views.

## NONRHEUMATOID DEFORMITIES

Nonrheumatoid deformity of the hand is less well understood by the radiologist than the orthopedic surgeon because the diagnosis is usually made on the basis of physical examination. Since much of the deformity is actually due to soft tissue abnormality, the radiographic examination is usually normal and is obtained only to exclude any associated bony abnormality. Mallet finger (baseball finger), described under fractures involving the hand, may also result from injury to the extensor tendon. The typical deformity consists of flexion at the distal interphalangeal joint and hyperextension at the proximal interphalangeal joint. This deformity may be teated by splinting as well as by operative repair. Trigger finger deformity results from swelling of the sublimis flexor tendon in a constricted sheath over a metacarpal head, producing an audible snap with flexion or extension resulting in eventual locking in flexion. Treatment is nonoperative for the acute phase and operative for the chronic stage. Gamekeeper's thumb, a nonrheumatoid deformity resulting from ulnar collateral ligament injury, is characterized by radial subluxation of the proximal phalanx of the thumb (Fig. 4–15). Radial stress views may be necessary to demonstrate the subluxation.

Dupuytren's contracture is a nonrheumatoid deformity resulting in flexion of the distal portion of the palm and fingers due to hypertrophy and contracture of the palmar aponeurosis. Flexion deformities, especially of the fourth and fifth fingers, may be observed radiographically. This entity is treated by soft tissue surgery. The carpal tunnel syndrome consists of compression of the median nerve between the flexor tendons and the transverse carpal ligaments (carpal tunnel). It is more commonly observed in middle-aged women. The syndrome may be bilateral, producing pain, numbness, and paresthesias in the distribution of the me-

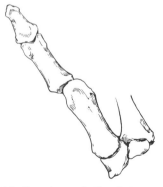

**Figure 4–15.** Gamekeeper's thumb is recognized by radial subluxation of the proximal phalanx and may require stress views for demonstration.

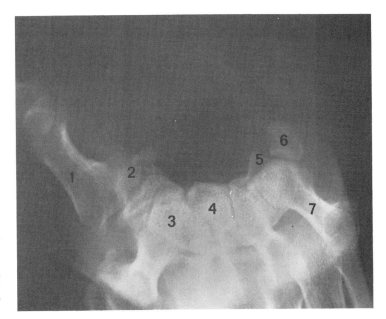

**Figure 4–16.** Carpal tunnel view. 1, First metacarpal; 2, trapezium; 3, scaphoid; 4, capitate; 5, hook of hamate; 6, pisiform; 7, fifth metacarpal.

dian nerve. There are many causes, and radiographs, including the carpal tunnel view, may demonstrate a bony etiology for compression, although most cases are due to soft tissue compression and demonstrate normal radiographs. The carpal tunnel view may demonstrate thickening of the soft tissues in the region of the carpal tunnel, deformity of the hook of the hamate, or calcium deposition in the carpal ligaments or flexor

tendons of the wrists, accounting for the carpal tunnel syndrome (Fig. 4–16). Treatment consists of soft tissue decompression.[25-29]

A ganglion is a cystic swelling in the region of a joint or tendon sheath, most commonly about the wrist. Radiographs are usually normal, and treatment consists of aspiration and injection or surgical excision.

Madelung deformity (Fig. 4–17) is char-

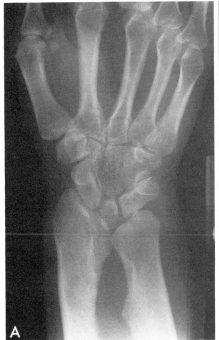

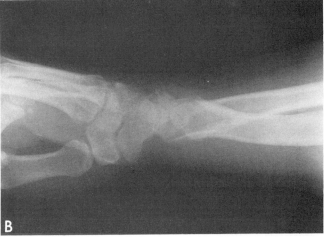

**Figure 4–17.** A and B, Madelung deformity. (Courtesy of Dr. Morrie Kricun, Philadelphia, Pennsylvania.)

acterized by shortening of the radius, and a V-shaped configuration between the distal radius and ulna and the proximal row of carpal bones on the anteroposterior projection. Excessive palmar tilting of the distal radius and dorsal dislocation of the distal ulna on the lateral view are also noted. This deformity is most commonly seen in females, developing at the time of puberty, and it is usually bilateral. A similar deformity may be seen in epiphyseal injury or infection.[30]

## RHEUMATOLOGIC PROBLEMS

Degenerative arthritis of the distal radioulnar joint is characterized radiographically by irregularity, sclerosis, narrowing, and spur formation of the distal ulna. Treatment consists of surgical removal of the distal ulna. Degenerative arthritis of the greater multangular–first metacarpal joint may be treated by arthrodesis or by an implant arthroplasty in which the greater multangular is removed and replaced by a silicone rubber implant (Fig. 4–18). The main complication of this type of arthroplasty is subsequent dislocation.[31].

Rheumatoid deformity of the hand and wrist results from muscle and tendon imbalance. This may be treated by soft tissue surgery, arthrodesis, or implant arthroplasty in order to relieve the pain and deformity. The deformities encountered include ulnar deviation at the metacarpophalangeal joints due to intrinsic muscle (interossei and lumbricals) and extensor tendon imbalance, boutonnière deformity or flexion of the proximal interphalangeal joint due to weakening or disruption of the extensor tendon, and swan-neck deformity consisting of hyperextension of the proximal interphalangeal joint and flexion of the metacarpophalangeal and distal interphalangeal joints owing to flexor tendon sheath synovitis (Fig. 4–19).

The soft tissue surgical procedures utilized in the management and treatment of rheumatoid deformity of the hand include synovectomy, tendon and muscle contracture release, and tendon transfer. Radiographically, improvement in alignment may

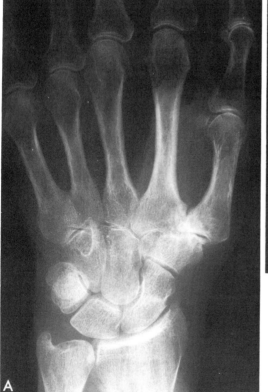

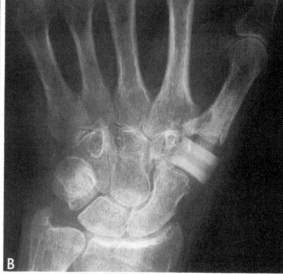

**Figure 4–18.** Degenerative arthritis of the greater multangular; first metacarpal joint *(A)*, treated by a silicone rubber implant *(B)*.

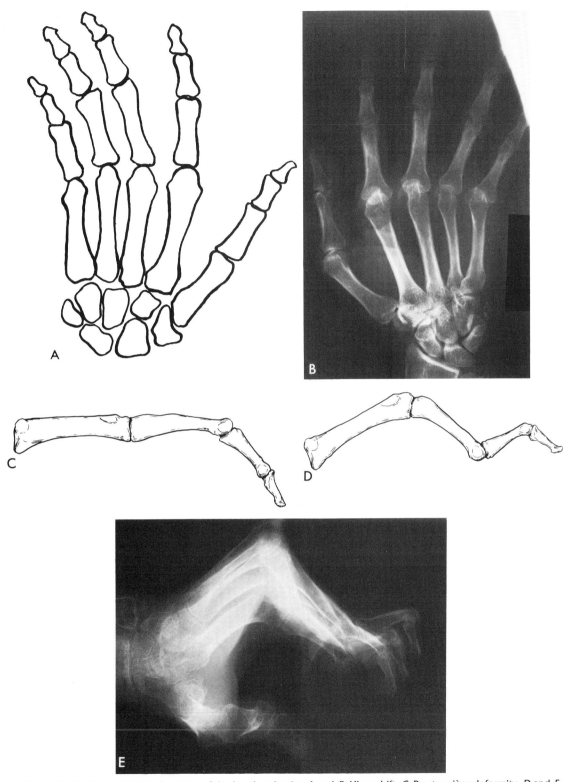

**Figure 4–19.** Rheumatoid deformities of the hand and wrist. *A* and *B*, Ulnar drift. *C*, Boutonnière deformity. *D* and *E*, Swan-neck deformity.

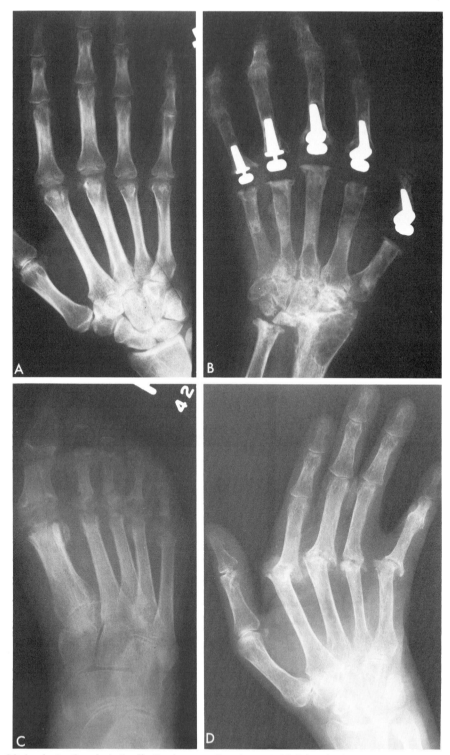

**Figure 4–20.** Implant arthroplasty is effective in correcting rheumatoid deformity in metacarpophalangeal (*A* to *C*) and metatarsophalangeal joints *(C)*. However, recurrent ulnar drift may occur as a complication *(D)*.

subsequently be observed. Implant arthroplasty utilizing a Silastic (Fig. 4–20 A) or metal (Fig. 4–20 B) prosthesis is effective in maintaining motion, correcting deformity, and providing stability to diseased metacarpophalangeal or metatarsophalangeal joints (Fig. 4–20 C). The metacarpal head is removed and the implant inserted into the medullary canal of the metacarpal and the phalanx. The implant is secured by the subsequent formation of a fibrous capsule. The possible complications of implant arthroplasty that may be evaluated radiographically include infection, dislocation, or fracture of the implant and recurrent ulnar drift (Fig. 4–20 D).[32, 33] Proximal interphalangeal joint disease is treated by arthrodesis.

More recently, radiocarpal implants have been utilized in the rheumatoid wrist, although these have not been as common as in the metacarpophalangeal joints. The flexible silicone rubber hinged implant, secured by fibrous encapsulation, and the rigid metallic total joint replacement, secured by methyl methacrylate, are the two main types of implants used (Fig. 4–21).

A resection arthroplasty (Darrach proce-

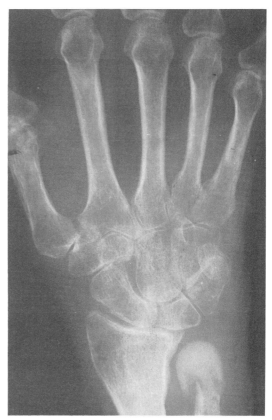

**Figure 4–22.** A resection arthroplasty of the distal ulna has been performed and a Silastic head implanted.

dure) or resection of less than 2 to 3 cm of the distal ulna may be performed because of pain. Instability and ulnar shift of the carpal bones may result but also may be prevented by an ulnar head implant (Fig. 4–22).

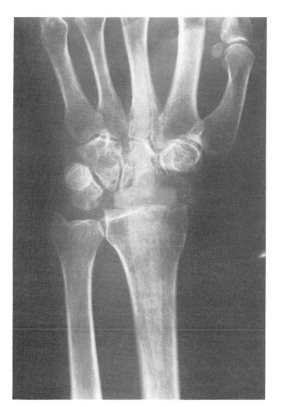

**Figure 4–21.** Total joint arthroplasty of the wrist.

## References

1. Genant HK, Kunoi D, Mall KD Sickles EA: Direct radiographic magnification for skeletal radiology. Radiology 123:47–55, 1977.
2. Brodeur AE: Microfocus direct magnification radiology in pediatric orthopedics and skeletal radiology. Orthop Review 3:91–98, 1979.
3. Frykman G: Fracture of the distal radius including sequelae-shoulder-hand-finger syndrome, disturbance in the distal radio-ulnar joint, and impairment of nerve function: a clinical and experimental study. Acta Orthop Scand 108:1–155, 1967.
4. Dowling JF, Sawyer B Jr: Comminuted Colle's fractures: evaluation of a method of treatment. J Bone Joint Surg 43A:657–668, 1961.
5. Parisien S: Settling in Colle's fracture: a review of the literature. Bull Hosp. Joint Dis 34:117–125, 1973
6. Ellis J: Smith's and Barton's fractures: a method of treatment. J Bone Joint Surg 47B:724–727, 1965.

7. Coleman HM: Injuries of the articular disc at the wrist. J Bone Joint Surg 42B:522–529, 1960.

8. Weigl K, Spira E: The triangular fibrocartilage of the wrist joint. Reconstr Surg Traumatol 11:139–153, 1969.

9. Meschan I: An Atlas of Anatomy Basic to Radiology. W. B. Saunders Co., Philadelphia, 1975, p. 108

10. Dobyns, JH, Linscheid, RL: Fractures and dislocations of the wrist. In Rockwood CA, Green DP: Fractures. Vol. 1. J. B. Lippincott, Co., Philadelphia, 1975 pp. 345–440

11. Mazet R Jr, Holh M: Fractures of the carpal navicular: analysis of ninety-one cases and review of the literature. J Bone Joint Surg 45A:82–112, 1963.

12. Russe O: Fractures of the carpal navicular: diagnosis, non-operative treatment, and operative treatment. J Bone Joint Surg 42A:759–768, 1960.

13. Verdan C: Fractures of the scaphoid. Surg Clin North Am 40:461–464, 1060.

14. McLaughlin HL: Fracture of the carpal navicular (scaphoid) bone: some observations based on treatment by open reduction and internal fixation. J Bone Joint Surg 36A:765–774, 1954.

15. Turek SL: The wrist. In Turek SL: Orthopaedics: Principles and their Applications. J.B. Lippincott, Philadelphia, 1978, pp. 972–993

16. Swanson AB: Silicone rubber implants for the replacement of the carpal scaphoid and lunate bones. Orthop Clin North Am 1:299–309, 1970.

17. Kaye JJ: Fractures and dislocations of the hand and wrist. Semin Roentgenol 13:109–116, 1978.

18. Swanson AB: Flexible Implant Resection Arthroplasty in the Hand and Extremities. C.V. Mosby, St. Louis, 1973.

19. Stark HH, Boyes JH, Wilson JN: Mallet finger. J Bone Joint Surg 44A:1061–1068, 1962.

20. Green DP, Rowland, SA: Fractures and dislocations of the hand. In Rockwood CA, Green DA: Fractures. Vol. 1. J.B. Lippincott Co., 1975, pp. 265–343

21. Kilbourne BC: Management of complicated hand fractures. Surg Clin North Am 48:201–213, 1968.

22. Kaye JJ: Fractures and dislocations of the hand and wrist. Semin Roentgenol 13:109–116, 1978

23. Green DP, Terry GC: Complex dislocation of the metacarpophalangeal joint: correlative pathological anatomy. J Bone Joint Surg 55A:1480–1486, 1973.

24. Sweterlitsch PR, Torg JS, Pollock H: Entrapment of a sesamoid in the index metacarpophalangeal joint: report of two cases. J Bone Joint Surg 51A:995–998, 1969

25. Carroll RE, Sinton W, Garcia A: Acute calcium deposits in the hand. JAMA 157:422–426, 1955

26. Phalen GS: Calcification adjacent to the pisiform bone. J Bone Joint Surg 34A:579–583, 1952.

27. Hart VL, Gaynor V: Roentgenographic study of the carpal canal J Bone Joint Surg 23:382–383, 1941.

28. Wilson JN: Profiles of the carpal canal. J Bone Joint Surg 36A:127–132, 1954.

29. Phalen GS: The carpal tunnel syndrome. J Bone Joint Surg 48A:211, 1966.

30. Edeiken J, Hodes PJ: Roentgen Diagnosis of Diseases of Bone. 2nd ed. Williams and Wilkins, Baltimore, 1970, pp. 109–110

31. Swanson AB: Disabling arthritis at the base of the thumb. J Bone Joint Surg 54A:456, 1972.

32. Adams JP, Neviaser, RJ: Complications of implant surgery in the hand. In Epps CH (ed): Complications in Orthopaedic Surgery. Vol. 2. J.B. Lippincott Co., Philadelphia, 1978, pp. 905–914

33. Granowitz S, Vainio K: Proximal interphalangeal joint arthrodesis in rheumatoid arthritis. Acta Orthop Scand 37:301, 1966.

# 5

# TRAUMA TO THE PELVIS

It is important to recognize bony injury to the pelvis, not because it necessitates extensive orthopedic surgery for correction but because of the relatively high morbidity and mortality accompanying the skeletal injury secondary to hemorrage or visceral trauma. Vehicular accidents and falls account for most of these significant injuries.

## RADIOLOGIC EVALUATION

In the suspected or obvious pelvis fracture, adequate delineation may be obtained by a standard anteroposterior view of the pelvis, both oblique projections, and a 30-degree cephalad angled projection to delineate the sacrum, since sacral fractures are frequently unrecognized owing to the contour of the sacrum as well as obscuration by feces and bowel (Fig. 5–1). If the injury includes trauma to the acetabulum, a 15 to 30 degree anterior oblique view will help to delineate the iliopubic column and posterior lip of the acetabulum, while a 30 to 45 degree posterior oblique view will help to delineate the ilioischial column and anterior acetabular rim fractures[1, 2] (see Table 5–1 and Fig. 5–2). Tomography has been useful in evaluating acetabular fractures, since size and number of major fracture fragments as

**Table 5–1.** PLAIN FILM EVALUATION OF TRAUMA TO THE PELVIS

1. AP pelvis
2. 15°–30° anterior oblique
3. 30°–45° posterior oblique
4. 30° cephalad angled projection

well as their position (anterior or posterior capsular space) can be ascertained; such information is very important to the orthopedic surgeon when planning the operative approach (Fig. 5–3). More recently, computerized tomography[3] has been helpful in demonstrating intra-articular fragments not well delineated on routine radiographs (Fig. 5–4). Close monitoring of the radiographic study by the radiologist is mandatory when dealing with trauma to the pelvis, since the study may be tailored according to the initial radiographic findings.

The analogy of the pelvis to a bony ring has long been recognized, as has the rule that a fracture or dislocation at one point in the ring must be accompanied by a disruption at another point in the ring, whether in the bone or at an articulation. At times, pubic rami fractures are observed following minor trauma without radiographic evidence of additional injury to the pelvis. In these cases symphysis pubis or sacroiliac joint separation must be suspected. More recently, this apparent isolated injury has been found to be associated with an obscured acetabular fracture or sacroiliac joint disruption, the first indication of which is on a bone scan. This further emphasizes the need for better delineation of the sacroiliac joints and the acetabulum in the patient with major or minor trauma to the pelvis who complains of hip or sacroiliac pain and of the usefulness of the radionuclide scan in delineating these subtle injuries.[4, 5] Whether the pelvis is subjected to major or minor trauma, it is again well to remember that if a fracture occurs at one site in the pelvic ring, an additional fracture or disruption

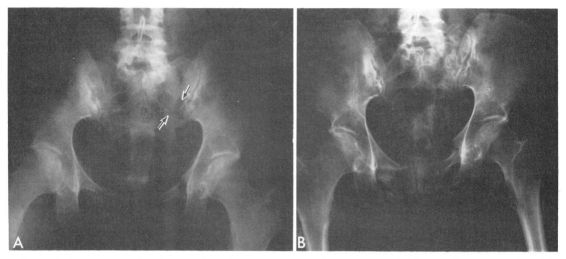

**Figure 5–1.** A sacral fracture is present *(A)* (arrows) but was not recognized until later *(B)*. Asymmetry of the left sacral ala and foramina is a clue to the presence of a sacral fracture. Bilateral pubic rami fractures are also present.

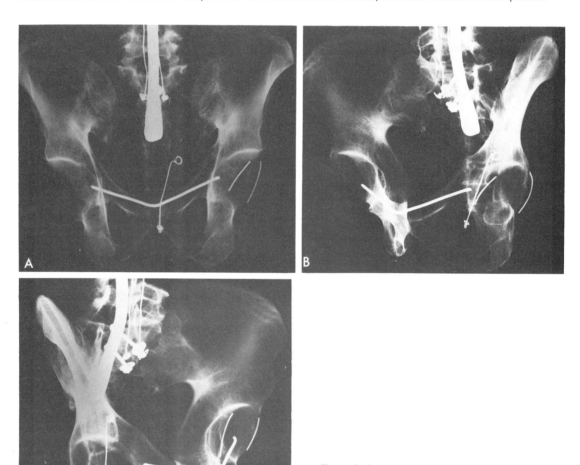

**Figure 5–2.** *A*, Anteroposterior view of the pelvis of a skeleton with anterior acetabular rim delineated by a short wire and the posterior acetabular rim delineated by the long wire. *B*, A 15 to 30 degree anterior oblique view delineating the iliopubic column and the posterior rim of the acetabulum. *C*, A 30 to 45 degree posterior oblique view delineating the ilioischial column and the anterior acetabular rim.

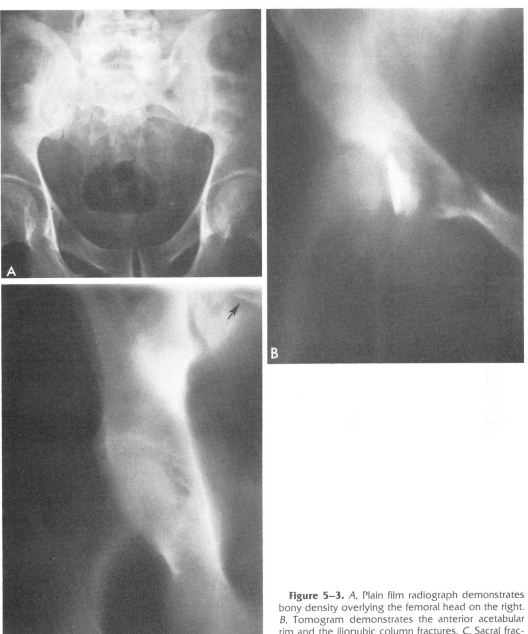

**Figure 5–3.** *A*, Plain film radiograph demonstrates bony density overlying the femoral head on the right. *B*, Tomogram demonstrates the anterior acetabular rim and the iliopubic column fractures. *C*, Sacral fracture was incidentally noticed and the tomographic field subsequently increased to include it as well (arrows).

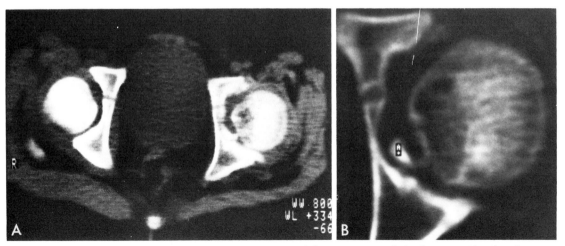

**Figure 5–4.** *A,* Computed tomography scan demonstrates a left posterior acetabular fracture with a free fragment in the joint space. *B,* Magnification view (× 2).

usually occurs at a more distant site. Pain over the symphysis pubis without demonstrable widening may be due to instability in the cephalocaudad direction. This instability may be demonstrated by erect views with individual weight-bearing on each leg (Fig. 5–5). Motion of the pubis up to 1.5 mm in the nonpregnant female and up to 0.5 mm in the male is normal. Movement of 2 mm or more causes symptoms and should provoke close scrutiny of the sacroiliac joint, which is frequently concomitantly involved and considerably more painful when affected by post-traumatic arthritis than by separation of the symphysis pubis.[6, 7]

Except for instances of direct trauma that may produce local fractures, injury of the symphysis is manifested by separation of or a change in the horizontal relationship of the two pubic bones or both. In normal individuals, the lower margin is a more reliable indicator of level than is the upper margin of the symphysis.

With a history of trauma, a slight offset of the inferior pubic margins should be regarded with suspicion. It is surprising, when this is appreciated, how often corresponding associated separation of a sacroiliac joint can be detected. Pelvic hematoma may be indicated on the plain film by displacement of the pelvic vein phleboliths (Fig. 5–6), but ultrasound and computed tomography may be helpful in evaluating hematoma in the pelvis [8, 12] (Table 5–2).

## ORTHOPEDIC-RADIOLOGIC CORRELATION

An understanding of the mechanism and classification of injury to the pelvis will aid in intelligent radiographic interpretation. A useful classification is presented in Table 5–3.[13]

**Table 5–3.** CLASSIFICATION OF PELVIC FRACTURES

Solitary fractures without discontinuity of the pelvic ring
  Avulsion fractures
    Anterior superior iliac spine
    Anterior inferior iliac spine
    Ischial tuberosity
  Fracture of the pubis or ischium
  Fracture of the wing of the ilium (Duverney)
  Fracture of the sacrum
  Fracture or dislocation of the coccyx
Discontinuity of the pelvic ring at a single site
  Fracture of two ipsilateral rami
  Fracture near or subluxation of the symphysis pubis
  Fracture near or subluxation of the sacroiliac joint
Discontinuity of the pelvic ring at two or more sites
  Bilateral pubic rami fractures (straddle fractures)
  Unilateral pubic rami fractures and fracture of the
    ilium or sacrum or sacroiliac dislocation (Malgaigne)
  Severe multiple fractures
Fractures of the acetabulum
  Undisplaced
  Displaced

**Table 5–2.** RADIOGRAPHIC EVALUATION OF PELVIC TRAUMA

1. Plain films
2. Tomography
3. Cystourethrography
4. Angiography
5. Ultrasound
6. CT scan

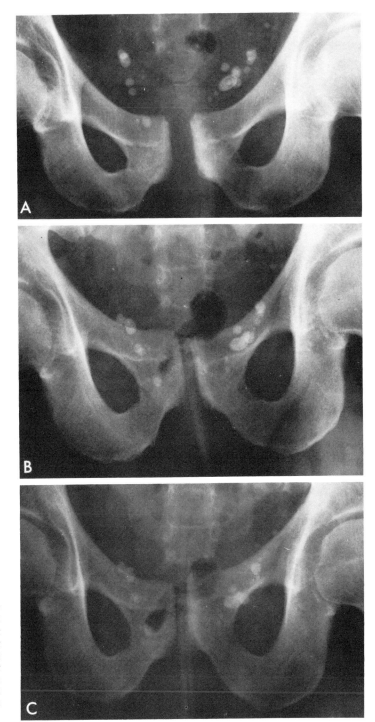

**Figure 5–5.** Cephalocaudad instability of the symphysis pubis is demonstrated by erect view with individual weight bearing on each leg. *A,* Erect weight bearing on both legs. *B,* Weight bearing on right leg. *C,* Weight bearing on left leg. Cephalocaudad motion greater than 1.5 mm in the nonpregnant female and greater than 0.5 mm in the male is abnormal.

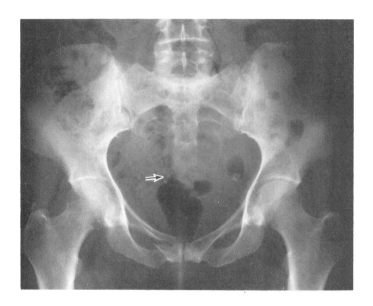

**Figure 5–6.** Phlebolith sign. Pelvic vein phleboliths on right are displaced medially by pelvic hematoma secondary to pubic fracture (arrow).

Treatment depends upon the stability of the fracture as well as whether or not dislocation is present. Mechanisms of injury, stability, and modes of treatment of various pelvic fractures are listed in Table 5–4.

Solitary fractures of the pelvis are characterized by their stability and rapid healing, with the exception of fractures of the coccyx, which are unstable. Avulsion fractures are commonly seen in athletic individuals. Often involved are the anterior superior iliac spine, due to hypercontraction of the sartorius muscle; the anterior inferior iliac spine, due to hypercontraction of the straight head of the rectus femoris muscle; and the ischial tuberosity, due to hypercontraction of the hamstrings (Figs. 5–7 to 5–9). A single fracture of the pubis or ischium is common in the elderly and may occur following a fall or as an insufficiency fracture in osteoporosis or osteomalacia.[14, 15] These fractures frequently present clinically as femoral neck fractures, necessitating a high index of suspicion and the use of additional views (obliques) (Fig. 5–10). Isolated fractures of the wing of the iliac bone, called Duverney fractures,[16] may occur (Fig. 5–11). Fractures of the sacrum frequently occur in association with other pelvic fractures and are frequently overlooked. The 30-degree cephalad angled anteroposterior projection will help in further delineation of these fractures, as will tomography.[17, 18] Coccyx fractures may produce chronic pain owing to their instability, and coccygectomy is recommended

by some.[19] Although disruption of the pelvic ring at one site only may occur, theoretically, since the pelvis is not a completely rigid ring in that the symphysis pubis and sacroiliac joint allow mobility, the stress is usually great enough to cause another fracture or subluxation or dislocation of the symphysis pubis or sacroiliac joint[20–23] (Fig. 5–12).

Discontinuity of the pelvic ring at two or more sites is approximately half as common as the stable fracture[24] and is usually associated with concomitant soft tissue injury. The Malgaigne fracture (Fig. 5–13) that is part of this group consists of unilateral fractures through the superior and inferior pubic rami and a fracture through the ilium or sacrum or a sacroiliac dislocation. It is an important entity to recognize because of the frequently associated cephalad displacement of the hip, resulting in shortening of the lower extremity and necessitating traction in its management.[25]

Severe multiple fractures of the pelvis result from greater forces applied to the pelvis and are associated, to a greater degree, with more severe hemorrhage and genitourinary injury.

Fractures of the acetabulum may be undisplaced or displaced, and may involve the rim or central portion of the acetabulum or, concomitantly, the ischium (ischioacetabular fracture of Walther). Approximately one third of the patients sustaining a pelvic fracture may have a concomitant acetabular frac-

*Text continued on page 91*

**Table 5–4.** MECHANISM OF INJURY, STABILITY, AND MODE OF TREATMENT OF PELVIC FRACTURES

| | Type of Fracture | Mechanism of Injury | Stability | Treatment |
|---|---|---|---|---|
| Single fractures of the pelvis | Avulsion Fractures | | | |
| | Anterior superior iliac spine | Sartorius | Stable | Bed rest |
| | Anterior inferior iliac spine | Rectus femoris | Stable | Bed rest |
| | Ischial tuberosity | Hamstrings | Stable | Bed rest |
| | Fracture of pubis or ischium | Elderly, insufficiency fractures | Stable | Bed rest |
| | Fracture of wing of ilium | Lateral compression force | Stable | Bed rest |
| | Fracture of sacrum | Direct trauma associated with multiple pelvic injuries | Stable | Bed rest |
| | Fracture or dislocation of coccyx | Falls in sitting position | Unstable, may cause persistent pain | Bed rest |
| Disruption of pelvic ring at one site | Fracture of two ipsilateral rami | Direct trauma, indirect trauma via femur | Stable | Bed rest |
| | Fracture near or subluxation of the symphysis pubis | Same | Stable | Bed rest |
| | Fracture near or subluxation of the sacroiliac joint | Same, associated with anterior ring fractures | Stable | Bed rest, pelvic sling or belt |
| Disruption of pelvic ring at two or more sites | Double vertical fractures and/or dislocation of the pubis (straddle fractures) | Crushing trauma, fall from heights, vehicular accidents | Unstable | Bed rest |
| | Double vertical fractures and/or dislocations (Malgaigne) | Same | Unstable | Lateral recumbency and/or plaster leg traction & pelvic hammock method |
| | Severe multiple fractures | Same | Unstable | Bed rest with or without sandbags, pelvic sling with extension |
| Fractures of the acetabulum | Undisplaced fracture | Crushing trauma, fall from heights, vehicular accidents | Stable | Bed rest |
| | Displaced fracture | Same | Unstable | Traction |

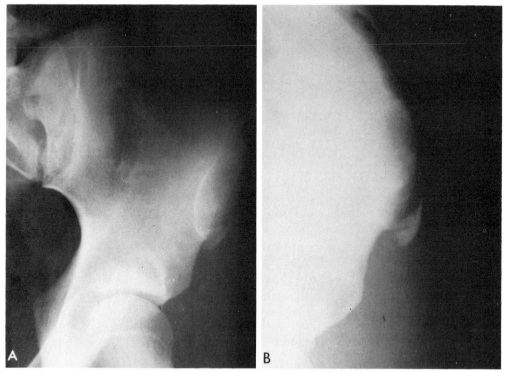

**Figure 5–7.** Avulsion fracture of the anterior superior iliac spine due to hypercontraction of the sartorius muscle. (Courtesy of Dr. G. W. Nixon, Salt Lake City, Utah.)

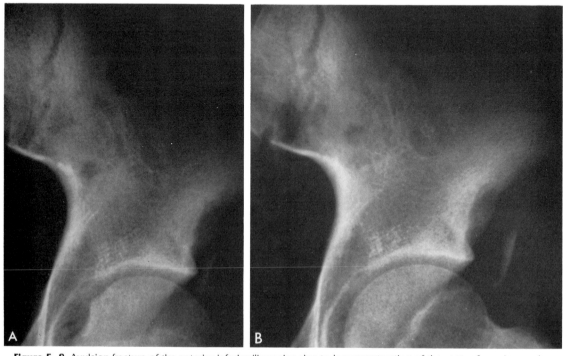

**Figure 5–8.** Avulsion fracture of the anterior inferior iliac spine due to hypercontraction of the rectus femoris muscle.

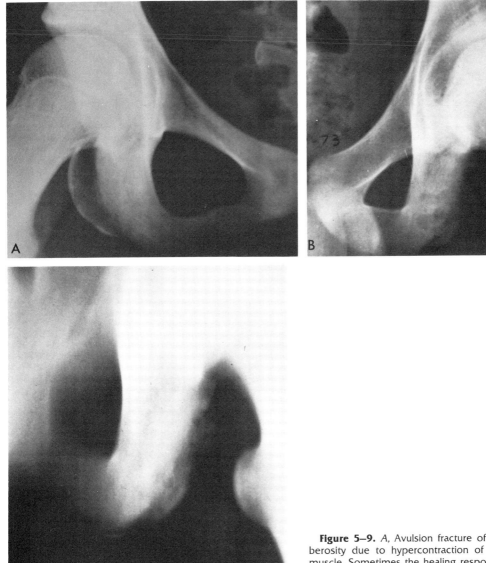

**Figure 5–9.** *A*, Avulsion fracture of the ischial tuberosity due to hypercontraction of the hamstring muscle. Sometimes the healing response may simulate a tumor such as a Ewing's sarcoma. *B*, Plain radiograph. *C*, Tomogram.

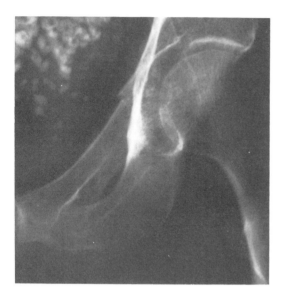

**Figure 5–10.** A left iliopubic ramus fracture is observed in an elderly female patient with chronic renal failure following minor trauma. The clinical suspicion was a femoral neck fracture.

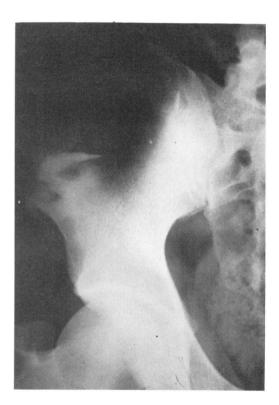

**Figure 5–11.** Isolated fracture of the wing of the iliac bone (Duverney fracture).

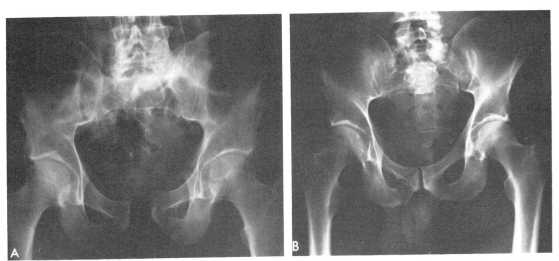

**Figure 5–12.** *A*, Diastasis of the symphysis pubis and right sacroiliac joint. *B*, Fracture of the right pubis and diastasis of the left sacroiliac joint.

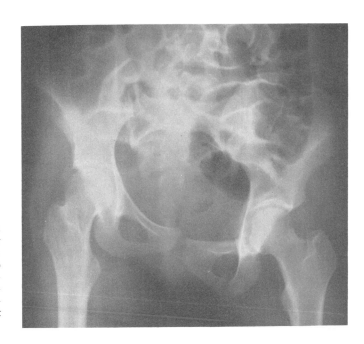

**Figure 5–13.** A Malgaigne fracture is characterized by an anterior and posterior pelvic ring fracture or dislocation which results in cephalad displacement of the hip and subsequent shortening. Note the cephalad displacement of the right hip, disruption of the right sacroiliac joint and symphysis pubis, and the fracture of the left ischiopubic junction.

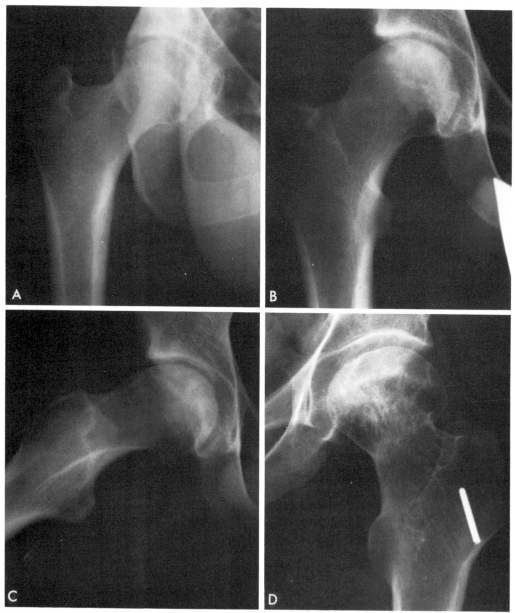

**Figure 5–14.** Posterior acetabular rim fracture was sustained on the right *(A)*, followed by avascular necrosis of the femoral head *(B* and *C)*. Intracapsular hematoma may cause compression of the vascular supply and subsequent avascular necrosis. *D,* Avascular necrosis after subcapital fracture on the left.

ture that is not recognized initially.[26] The importance of this is reflected in the corollary that femoral head damage may occur in displaced or undisplaced acetabular fractures (Fig. 5–14) owing to disruption of the blood supply with subsequent development of femoral head necrosis or osteoarthritis.[27, 28] When acetabular fractures are comminuted and many loose fragments are present, tomography or computed tomography allows the orthopedic surgeon to plan the operative approach, depending on the anterior or posterior intracapsular location of the bony fragments that must be removed or stabilized (see Fig. 5–4). A comminuted acetabular dome fracture most often means poor end result, necessitating arthroplasty (Fig. 5–15).

## COMPLICATIONS

The complications resulting from pelvic fractures, rather than the fractures themselves, account for the morbidity and mortality in these patients. The most important complications[29] include hemorrhage, bladder and urethral rupture, and neurologic damage to the sacral nerves (Table 5–5). Hemorrhage, the most serious complication because it is life threatening, is common

**Table 5–5.** COMPLICATIONS OF PELVIC FRACTURES

| |
| --- |
| Hemorrhage |
| Bladder or urethral rupture |
| Neurologic damage |

because of the close proximity of major blood vessels and rich venous plexuses surrounding the rectum, vagina, bladder, and prostate. Spontaneous hemostasis usually occurs following stabilization and reduction of pelvic fractures. Pelvic angiography and venography are useful in localizing the source of bleeding in those cases of persistent hemorrhage.[30, 31, 32] Control of persistent bleeding by surgical ligation is difficult and frequently unsuccessful, whereas balloon catheterization or selective arterial embolization (Fig. 5–16) has been employed successfully.[33, 34, 35]

Urethral bladder injuries have a higher incidence in patients with symphysis pubic separation or pubic rami fractures. The posterior urethra is most commonly ruptured. This injury is limited to the male because of the short mobile urethra in the female. Because an already traumatized urethra may be further damged by attempts at passing a Foley catheter to perform a cystogram, a retrograde urethrogram should be performed

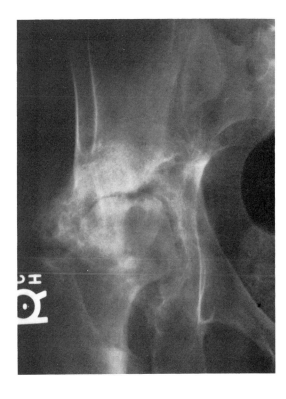

**Figure 5–15.** The markedly comminuted fracture of the acetabular dome has healed but, as frequently occurs, post-traumatic arthritis had developed.

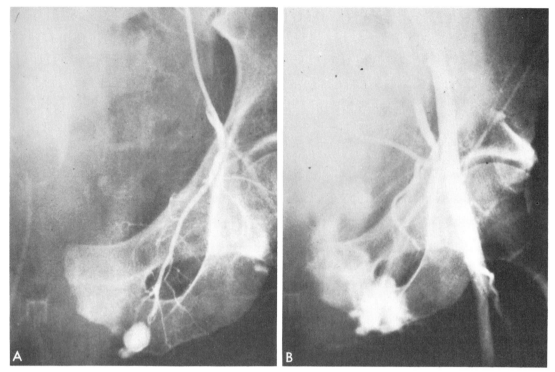

**Figure 5–16.** Laceration of the pudendal branch of the internal iliac artery was controlled by embolization with Gelfoam. *A*, Angiogram demonstrating pudendal artery laceration. *B*, Angiogram after embolization with Gelfoam.

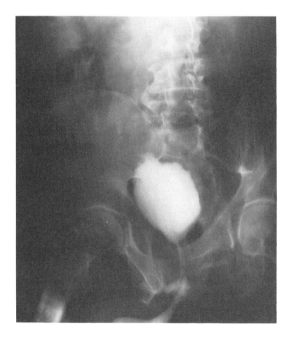

**Figure 5–17.** Posterior urethral rupture secondary to pelvic trauma demonstrated on a retrograde urethrogram.

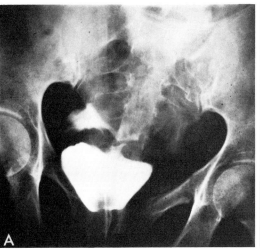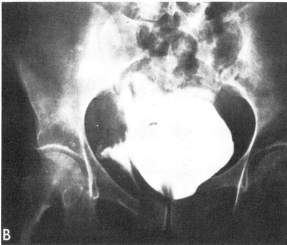

**Figure 5–18.** Retrograde cystogram demonstrating *(A)* intraperitoneal and *(B)* extraperitoneal urinary bladder rupture. Contrast media outlining bowel loops indicates an intraperitoneal rupture, whereas extravasation of contrast media confined around the urinary bladder demonstrates an extraperitoneal rupture.

prior to the cystogram to exclude the possibility of a urethral tear (Fig. 5–17). Rupture of the bladder represents the major urinary tract injury in the female and may be intraperitoneal or extraperitoneal. Retrograde cystourethrography in the male and cystography in the female should be performed to exclude lower urinary tract injury (Fig. 5–18).[33, 36, 37]

# References

1. Armbuster TG, Guerra J Jr, Resnick D, Georgen TG, Feingold ML, Niwayama G, Danzig LA: The adult hip: an anatomic study. Radiology 128:1–10, 1978
2. Judet R, Judet J, Letournel E: Fractures of the acetabulum: classification and surgical approaches for open reduction. J Bone Joint Surg 46A:1615–1646, 1964
3. Gilula LA, Murphy WA, Tailor CC, Patel RB: Computed tomography of the osseous pelvis. Radiology 132:107–114, 1979
4. Pearson JR, Hargadon EJ: Fracture of the pelvis involving the floor of the acetabulum. J Bone Joint Surg 44B:550, 1962
5. Gertzbein SD, Chenoweth DR: Occult injuries of the pelvic ring. Clin. Orthop 128:202–207, 1977
6. Taylor RG: Pelvic dislocations. Br J Surg 30:126–132, 1942
7. Chamberlain WE: The symphysis pubis in the roentgen examination of the sacroiliac joint. AJR 24:621–625, 1930
8. Steinbach HL: Identification of pelvic masses by phlebolith displacement. AJR 83:1063–1066, 1960
9. Fenlon JW, Augustin C: The significance of pelvic phlebolith displacement. J Urol 106:595–598, 1971
10. Levitt RG, Sagel SS, Stanley RJ, Evens RG: Computed tomography of the pelvis. Semin Roentgenol 13:193–211, 1978
11. McLeod RA, Stephens DH, Beabout JW, Sheedy PF II, Hattery RR: Computed tomography of the skeletal system. Semin Roentgenol 13:235–247, 1978
12. Redman HC: Computed tomography of the pelvis. Radiol Clin NAM 15:441–448, 1977
13. Kane WJ: Fractures of the pelvis. In Rockwood CA, Green DP: Fractures. J.B. Lippincott Co., Philadelphia, 1975, p. 905–1011
14. Garcia A Jr: Fractures of the pelvis. In Bick EM (ed): Trauma in the Aged. McGraw-Hill, New York, 1960
15. Hauser CW, Perry JF Jr: Massive hemorrhage from pelvic fractures. Minnesota Med 49:285–290, 1966
16. Peltier LF: Complications associated with fractures of the pelvis. J Bone Joint Surg 47A:1060–1069, 1965
17. Furey WW: Fractures of the pelvis with special reference to associated fractures of the sacrum. AJR 47:89–96, 1942
18. Medelman JP: Incidence of associated fractures of the sacrum. AJR 42:100–103, 1939
19. Watson-Jones R: Fractures and Joint Injuries. Williams and Wilkins, Baltimore, 1957
20. Bertin EJ: Separation of the symphysis pubis. AJR 30:797–803, 1933
21. Forsee GG: Clinical observations of pelvic fractures. Am J Surg 38:145–149, 1924
22. Watson-Jones R: Dislocations and fracture-dislocations of the pelvis. Br J Surg 25:773–781, 1938
23. McLaughlin HL: Fractures of the hips. In Moseley HF (ed): Accident Surgery. Vol. 2. Appleton-Century-Crofts, New York, 1964
24. Dunn W, Morris HD: Fractures and dislocations of the pelvis. J Bone Surg 50A:1639–1648, 1968
25. Malgaigne JF: Treatise on Fractures. J.B. Lippincott, Co., Philadelphia, 1859
26. Pearson JR, Hargadon EJ: Fractures of the pelvis involving the floor of the acetabulum. J Bone Joint Surg 44B:550–561, 1962

27. Elliott RB: Central fractures of the acetabulum. Clin Orthop 7:189–201, 1956
28. Eichenholtz SN, Stark RN: Central acetabular fractures. J Bone Surg 46A:695–714, 1964
29. Looser KG, Crombrie HD Jr: Pelvic fractures: an anatomic guide to severity of injury. Review of 100 cases. Am J Surg 132:638–642, 1976
30. Athanasoulis CA: Angiography to assess pelvic vascular injury. New Engl J Med 284:1329, 1971
31. Margolies MN, Ring EJ, Waltman AC, Kerr WS Jr, Braun S: Arteriography in the management of hemorrhage from pelvic fractures. New Engl J Med, 287:317–321, 1972
32. Reynolds BM, Balsano NA: Venography in pelvic fractures. A clinical evaluation. Ann Surg 173:104–106, 1971
33. Monahan PRW, Taylor RG: Dislocation and fracture-dislocation of the pelvis. Injury 6:325–333, 1975
34. Sheldon GF, Winestock DP: Hemorrhage from open pelvic fracture controlled intraoperatively with balloon catheter. J Trauma 18:68–70, 1978
35. vanYork H, Perilberger RR, Muller H: Selective arterial embolization for control of traumatic pelvic hemorrhage. Surgery 83:133–137, 1978
36. Flaherty JJ, Kelley R, Burnett B, Bucy J, Surian M, Schildkraut D, Clarke BG: Relationship of pelvic bone fracture patterns to injuries of urethra and bladder. J Urol 99:297–300, 1968
37. Trafford HS: Types of fractures of the pelvis with associated urethral ruptures and relative frequency. Postgrad Med J 34:656–657, 1958

# 6

# THE HIP AND FEMUR

## TRAUMA TO THE HIP

### Femoral Neck Fractures

Femoral neck fractures occur most commonly in the older patient. If intracapsular, they may be associated with avascular necrosis due to traumatic disruption or compression of the blood supply by intracapsular hematomas. The greater the degree of fracture displacement, the higher the incidence of complicating avascular necrosis, which may not become evident for several years after the injury.[1] The earliest radiographic features of this complication consist of increased bone density or flattening of the weight-bearing portion (supralateral aspect) of the articular surface of the femoral head (Fig. 6–1).[2] Since femoral neck fractures may commonly exhibit delayed healing or nonunion requiring prolonged bed rest, operative internal fixation is usually employed so that the patient can be mobilized early and complications therefore minimized. Modalities more recently cited as useful in detecting avascular necrosis or nonunion prior to radiographic changes include radionuclide scanning and perosseous venography.[3, 4] Normally, radionuclide activity should decrease by four months after femoral neck fracture; if it increases at the fracture site 6 to 18 months postfracture, nonunion is suggested.

Radionuclide scanning, utilizing $^{99m}$TcSc (technetium sulfur colloid), is most effective in detecting early avascular necrosis immediately after fracture and prior to plain film change and should show decreased activity. This information will aid the orthopedic surgeon in deciding whether or not to perform a bone graft or muscle pedicle graft. If the bone scan is obtained somewhat later, its value in detecting avascular necrosis is less, since it may show increased activity secondary to repair that occurs following avascular necrosis. It is at this time that a plain film is very helpful. (Fig. 6–2). With respect to perosseous venography, if extraosseous draining veins are visualized following direct injection of the femoral head, viability (nonsignificant avascular necrosis) of the femoral head is demonstrated, whereas if the contrast medium pools in the fracture site, significant avascular necrosis and therefore nonviability of the femoral head is concluded. At present, radionuclide scanning has been more widely accepted and used than perosseous venography.

### Internal Fixation of Femoral Neck Fractures

Internal fixation of femoral neck fractures may be accomplished by the following:

**Multiple Pins.** Hagie, Knowles, or Steinmann pins may be used as well as Deyerle pins, in which case a metal template secures the pins, allowing them to slide and cause impaction (Fig. 6–3).

**Fixed Nail (Smith-Peterson, Jewett) or Screw.** These provide fixation while positioned in valgus along the calcar, with the tip within 1 cm of the subchondral bone.

**Sliding Nail or Screw.** These fixation devices provide better impaction of the fracture fragments due to their sliding capability (Fig. 6–4) and reduce the chance of perforation

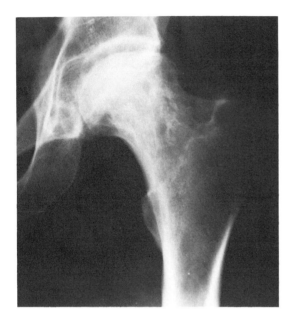

**Figure 6–1.** Avascular necrosis of the femoral head following a femoral neck fracture that healed is indicated by cystic and sclerotic changes as well as mild flattening of the femoral head. Preservation of the joint space is important in distinguishing this entity from degenerative arthritis.

through the femoral head. The barrel containing the nail or screw should not cross the fracture site and the nail or screw should extend to just below and not through the subchondral bone. A bone graft may be done at the time of internal fixation to promote stabilization and union of the fracture as well as vascularization of the femoral head.[5, 6] Quadratus femoris muscle pedicle bone grafts obtained from the posterior surface of the femur are transferred to the fracture site with an intact blood supply and screwed in place.[7]

**Complications of Internal Fixation.** Complications of internal fixation (see Fig. 1–15) include inadequate reduction or fixation as well as bending or fracturing of the fixation device.[8]

**Endoprosthesis.** Both the Austin-Moore and Thompson endoprostheses (Fig. 6–5) consist of a vitallium femoral head and an intramedullary stem. The Austin-Moore prosthesis is distinguished by fenestrations in the superior portion of the stem through which bone growth occurs, providing greater stability. Complications observed with these

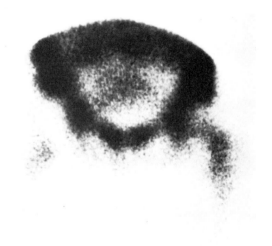

**Figure 6–2.** Radionuclide scan demonstrating avascular necrosis of the femoral head on the right. There is decreased activity in the right femoral head early post–femoral neck fracture. (Courtesy of Dr. F. Datz, University of Utah Medical Center, Salt Lake City, Utah.)

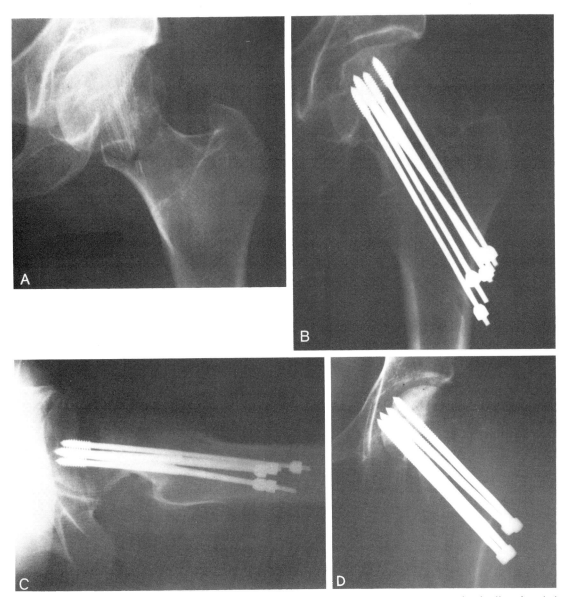

**Figure 6–3.** *A* to *C*, Knowles pin fixation of a femoral neck fracture. *D*, Penetration of the joint by the Knowles pin is a complication necessitating correction in order to avoid the induction of arthritis.

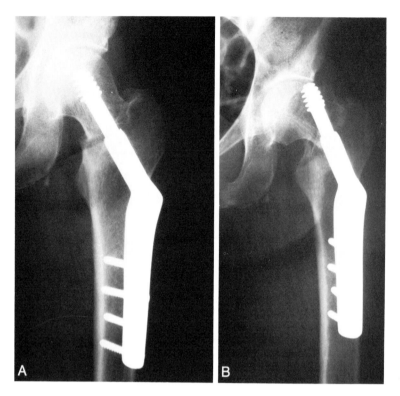

**Figure 6–4.** Sliding nail fixation of a femoral neck fracture with subsequent slippage of the nail and varus deformity.

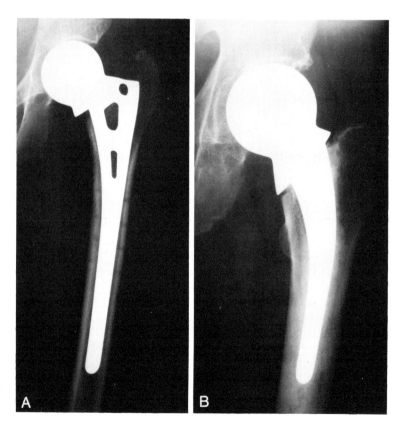

**Figure 6–5.** *A,* Austin-Moore prosthesis. *B,* Thompson prosthesis.

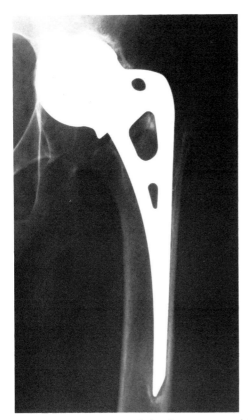

**Figure 6–6.** Protrusio acetabulae is a common late complication of the endoprosthesis. Note the lucent zone adjacent to the inferior tip of the prosthesis due to resorption of bone secondary to loosening.

endoprostheses include disintegration of the calcar and subsequent sinking of the prosthesis, protrusio acetabulae due to thinning of the medial portion of the acetabular roof (Fig. 6–6), loosening, or breakage of the prosthesis.[9, 10, 11]

These prostheses are primarily utilized in the elderly patient, in whom early weight-bearing is particularly important and whose physical activity will be limited.

## Intertrochanteric Fractures

Stability of the intertrochanteric fracture depends upon abutment of the medial femoral cortex against the cortex of the calcar. When this does not occur, as in comminuted fractures, an unstable fracture exists. The stable intertrochanteric fracture is treated by a fixed nail or screw, the tip of which should be within 1 cm of the subchondral cortex, and a side plate, which should be secured to both femoral cortices. The unstable inter-

trochanteric fracture is treated with a sliding screw or nail that allows impaction of the cortical fragments in the region of the calcar, and in so doing provides stability. Medial femoral shaft displacement prior to internal fixation (Fig. 6–7) may also be performed to increase stability and decrease the incidence of varus deformity. This increased medial displacement should be recognized as intentional rather than due to slippage or poor reduction.[12–16]

**Complications of Intertrochanteric Fractures.** Complications of treatment include (Fig. 6–8): internal fixation device failure with resulting coxa vara deformity, penetration of the femoral head by the internal fixation device with subsequent development of traumatic arthritis, loosening of the side plate screws, and metal fatigue.[8]

## Subtrochanteric Fractures

Subtrochanteric fractures require alignment of the medial femoral cortex for stability. This is achieved by open reduction and internal fixation. The Zickel nail, an effective fixation device for this type of fracture, consists of a short intramedullary rod with a proximal perforation, allowing transfixion by a nail into the femoral neck. A rigid relationship is maintained between the nail and the intramedullary rod.

**Complications of Subtrochanteric Fractures.** Complications of treatment include delayed union, nonunion, and failure of the fixation device to maintain reduction.[8]

## Fractures of the Femoral Shaft

Fractures of the femoral shaft require different fixation, depending upon their location. Those in the midportion of the shaft where the diameter is relatively constant and hence good intramedullary fixation is achieved, are treated by intramedullary rods (Ender, Kuntscher, or Rush rod) or by a sideplate and screws if extensive comminution is present (Fig. 6–9). Fractures at either end of the shaft necessitate plates and screws for fixation because of deforming muscle attachments and the ineffectiveness of the intramedullary rod in these expanded regions (Fig. 6–10). Fractures of the mid and distal femoral shaft may be treated with a

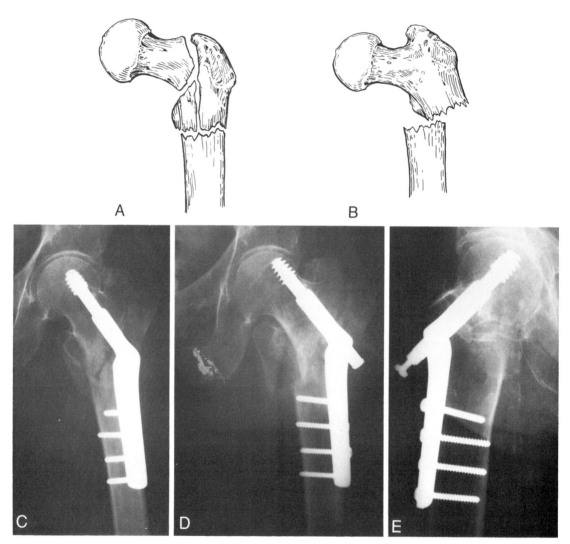

**Figure 6–7.** *A* and *B*, Intentional medial displacement of the distal femoral fracture fragment prevents accentuated varus deformity. *C* and *D*, Interval slippage medially of the distal fracture fragment has occurred with resulting impaction and further stability of the fracture. *E*, Excessive medial displacement has occurred with marked varus deformity resulting instead of penetration of the femoral head by the screw.

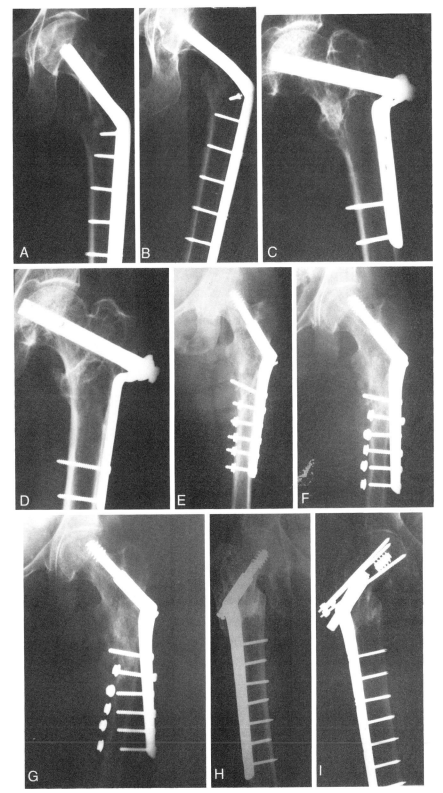

**Figure 6–8.** Complications of the intertrochanteric fracture include the following: *A* and *B*, Coxa vara deformity. *C* and *D*, Intra-articular penetration by fixation device. *E* to *G*, Loosening of side plate screws. *H* and *I*, Metal fatigue of the hardware.

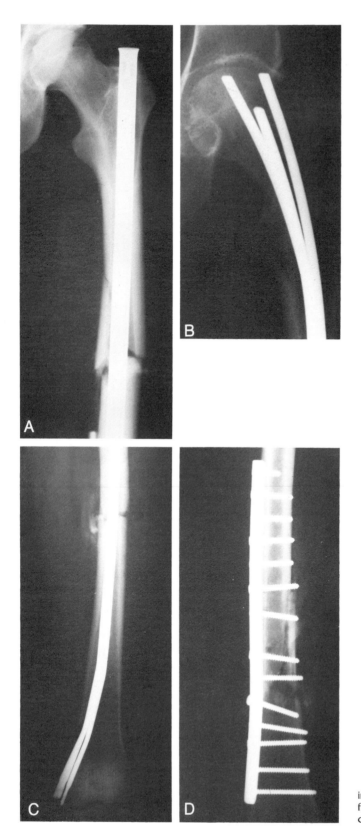

**Figure 6–9.** Ender *(A)* and Rush *(B* and *C)* intramedullary rod fixation of a femoral shaft fracture. *D,* Side plate and screw fixation of a comminuted femoral shaft fracture.

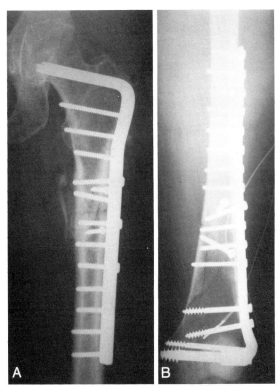

**Figure 6–10.** Plate and screw fixation is required for proximal *(A)* or distal *(B)* femoral shaft fractures since the intramedullary rod would not provide adequate immobilization in these expanded regions.

cast brace, which allows the muscles to exert a hydrodynamic stabilizing effect on the fracture and also allows early mobilization (see Fig. 1–2).[17] If angulation occurs, it can be corrected by wedging of the cast. Skin and skeletal traction may also be used in the management of femoral fractures.

**Complications of Treatment of Femoral Shaft Fractures.** Complications of treatment of femoral shaft fractures by intramedullary nailing include entry of the nail into the knee joint or excessive protrusion above the greater trochanter causing a bursitis, bending of the nail resulting from weakening of the metal, delayed union, nonunion, or osteomyelitis (Fig. 6–11). Migration of the nail may result from motion at the fracture site. Compression plate and screw fixation may be complicated by compression plate breakage (see Fig. 1–16).[18, 19]

## ARTHRITIS OF THE HIP

Degenerative or post-traumatic arthritis of the hip may be approached surgically in different ways, depending on the age of the patient and the severity of the arthritis.

### Osteotomy

The purpose of the osteotomy is to make the articular surfaces more congruent and distribute the stresses over a wider area of the joint (Figs. 6–12 and 6–13). It is used in the early stage of the disease in younger patients. The type of osteotomy performed depends upon the specific clinical and physical findings (see Table 6–1). The radiograph is used in assessing the degree of healing of the osteotomy as well as the more common complications, such as nonunion and infection.[32]

### Cup Arthroplasty

A vitallium (chromium-cobalt-molybdenum alloy) cup is fitted over the femoral head (Fig. 6–14). This is utilized mainly in younger patients.

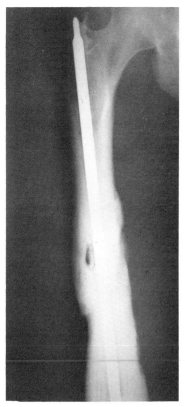

**Figure 6–11.** Complications of treatment of femoral shaft fractures include osteomyelitis, indicated radiographically by exuberant cortical sclerosis and central lucency.

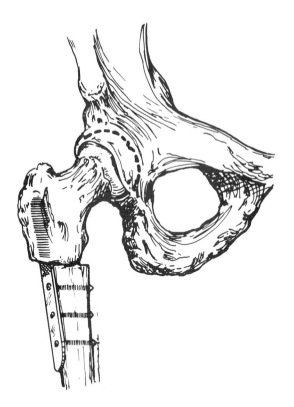

**Figure 6–12.** A McMurray medial displacement oste-otomy may be performed to redistribute the stress of weight bearing over a wider area of the joint.

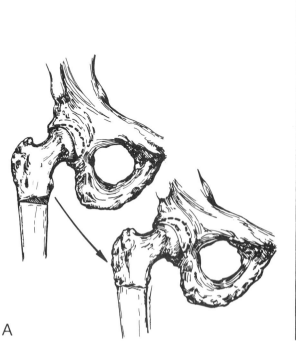

A

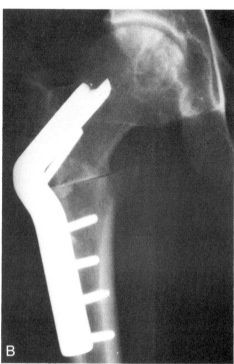

B

**Figure 6–13.** Legend on opposite page.

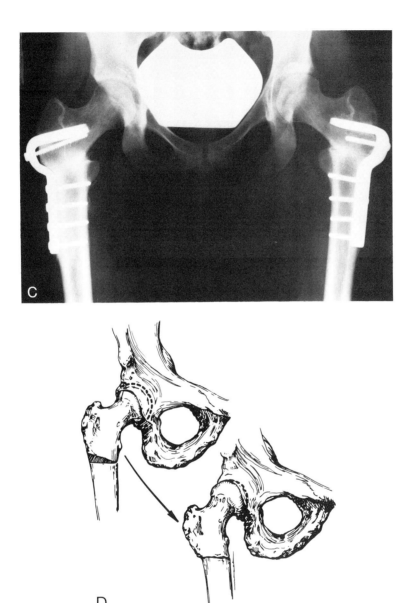

**Figure 6–13.** *A*, Varus osteotomy. A medially oriented wedge of bone is removed to allow the hip to go into varus and the head of the femur to rotate medially into the acetabulum. *B*, Varus osteotomy for avascular necrosis. *C*, Bilateral varus osteotomies for anteversion. *D*, Valgus osteotomy. Laterally oriented wedge of bone is removed to allow the hips to go into valgus and the head of the femur to rotate laterally out of the acetabulum.

**Table 6–1.** CONDITIONS REQUIRING
OSTEOTOMY PROCEDURES

| Condition | Osteotomy Procedure |
|---|---|
| Osteoarthritis | Varus or valgus proximal femoral osteotomy |
| Slipped capital femoral epiphysis | Proximal femoral osteotomy |
| Coxa vara | Proximal femoral osteotomy |
| Femoral torsion or anteversion | Proximal or distal femoral osteotomy |
| Fracture malunion | Femoral shaft osteotomy |
| Genu varum or valgum | Supracondylar (distal femoral) osteotomy |

## Total Hip Arthroplasty

Total hip arthroplasty is performed in older individuals with osteoarthritis, rheumatoid arthritis, or ankylosing spondylitis; in instances of previously failed endoprosthesis, cup arthroplasty, or osteotomy; and in certain resectable tumors of the proximal femur. The acetabular component of the prosthesis is made of high-density polyethylene with a metal marker ring, while the femoral component is a metal alloy (Fig. 6–15A). Original total hip components were Charnley-Mueller and Turner-Aufranc types, which could be identified radiographically by the femoral head sitting centrally in the acetabular component of the Charnley-Mueller type and eccentrically in the Turner-Aufranc type (Fig. 6–15). Since then, modifications of these hip replacement types have been made. In addition to implantation of an acetabular and femoral component, a greater trochanteric osteotomy may or may not be performed to allow wider surgical exposure of the hip.

The ideal position of the acetabular component is 45 degrees of abduction and 10 to 15 degrees of anteversion (Fig. 6–16A). Whether or not the acetabular component is anteverted or retroverted is determined from the groin lateral view (Fig. 6–16B). The femoral component is implanted in a valgus position, which is indicated by alignment of the femoral stem along the medial femoral cortex. Malpositioning of the acetabular component may result in recurrent dislocation if the cup is excessively vertical or retroverted, or in limited abduction of the hip if it is excessively horizontal (Figs. 6–17 and 6–18). When dislocation does occur, it is most commonly posterior in direction

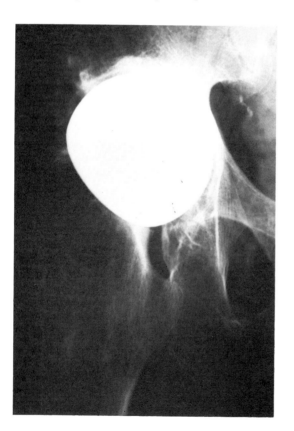

**Figure 6–14.** Cup arthroplasty.

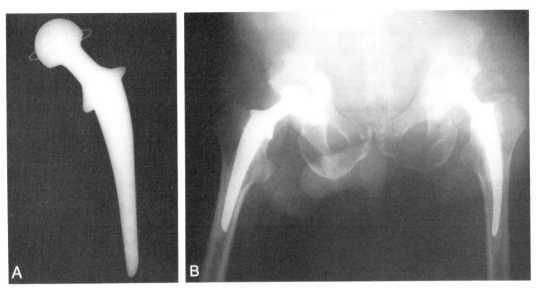

**Figure 6–15.** *A,* Radiograph of total hip replacement components. The polyethylene portion of the acetabular component becomes radiographically visible if surrounded by barium-impregnated methylmethacrylate. *B,* Charnley-Mueller (left) and Turner au Franc (right) prostheses.

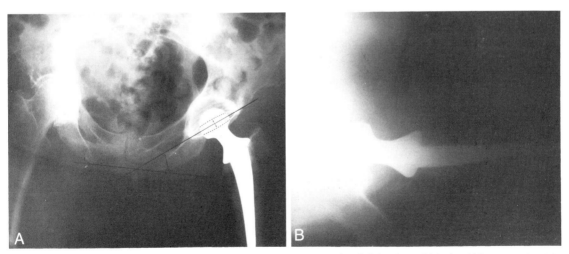

**Figure 6–16.** *A,* Important acetabular measurements include the angle of abduction, which should be approximately 45 degrees (large arrow), and the angle of anteversion, which should be approximately 10 to 15 degrees (small arrow). *B,* The groin lateral view is necessary to distinguish anteversion from retroversion of the acetabular component.

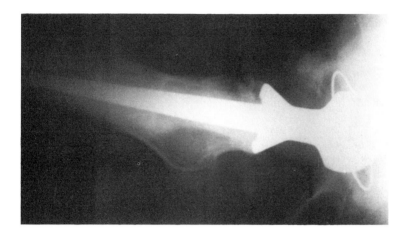

**Figure 6–17.** Retroversion of the acetabular component.

(Fig. 6–19). Malpositioning of the femoral component resulting in a lack of valgus allows the femoral stem to act as a stress-riser on the immediately adjacent bone, which may result in fracture (Fig. 6–20). Fracture may occur not only in the adjacent bone but also through the stem of the femoral component owing to metal fatigue or through the methyl methacrylate (Fig. 6–21). Heterotopic bone, although a complication of total hip arthroplasty, is usually asymptomatic and not significant. At times, it may cause limitation of range of motion; however, the physical examination rather than the radiograph is more accurate in determining this (Fig. 6–22). Heterotopic bone occurs with increased incidence in patients with ankylosing spondylitis following total hip replacement (Fig. 6–23).

Normally, a lucent zone 1 to 2 mm in width may develop at the methacrylate-bone interface. If this zone is greater than 1 to 2 mm, or if it is irregular or scalloped in contour, or if there is a lucent zone at the

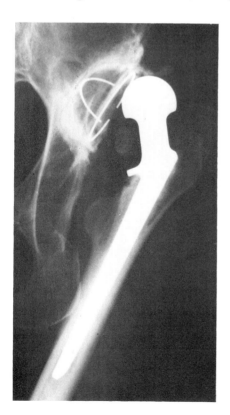

**Figure 6–18.** Excessive vertical axis of the acetabular component will predispose to dislocation.

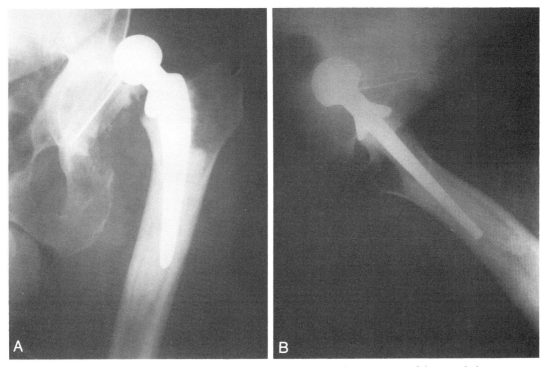

**Figure 6–19.** Posterior dislocation of the femoral component because of retroversion of the acetabular component. *A,* Anteroposterior view. *B,* Lateral view (same patient as in Fig. 6–17).

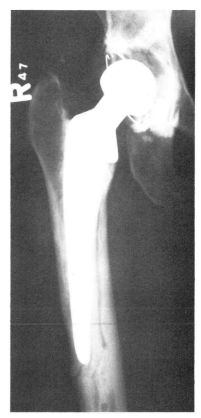

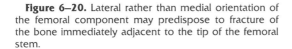

**Figure 6–20.** Lateral rather than medial orientation of the femoral component may predispose to fracture of the bone immediately adjacent to the tip of the femoral stem.

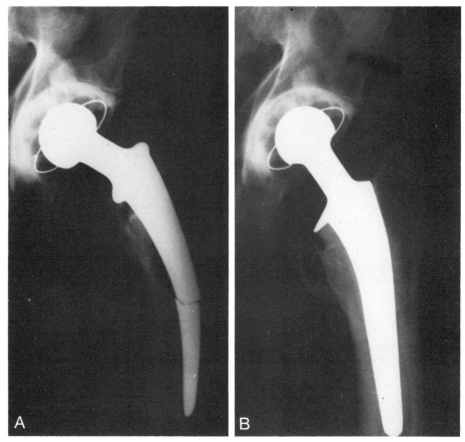

**Figure 6–21.** Metal fatigue resulting in fracture through the femoral stem *(A)* necessitating revision *(B)*.

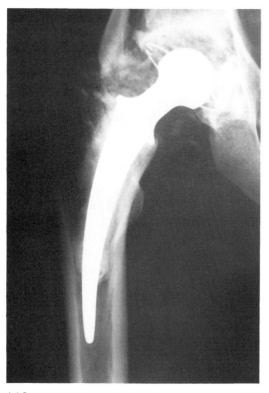

**Figure 6–22.** Radiograph demonstrating marked heterotopic bone formation. The patient had full range of motion, however.

110

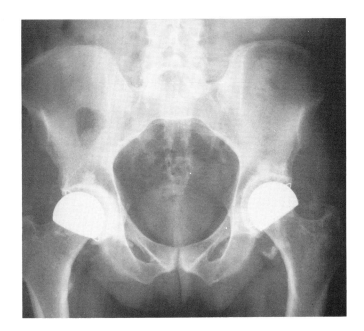

**Figure 6–23.** Patient with ankylosing spondylitis and heterotopic bone formation bilaterally.

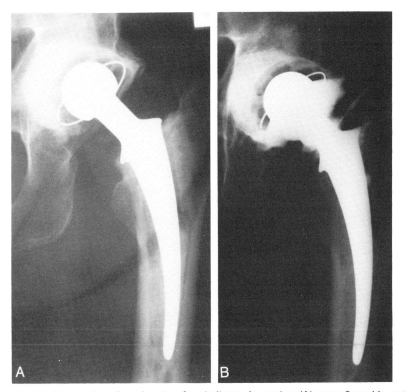

**Figure 6–24.** Lucency at the metal-methacrylate interface indicates loosening *(A)* as confirmed by arthrography *(B).*

**Table 6–2.** IMPORTANT PLAIN FILM FINDINGS OF TOTAL HIP PROSTHESES

Angle of abduction 45°
Angle of anteversion 10°–15°
Lucent zones: Bone–Cement
Cement–Prosthesis
Alignment of femoral stem

metal-methacrylate interface (Fig. 6–24), these constitute the plain film findings of loosening although loosening may not always be present.[20, 21] Loosening is the most frequent cause of prosthetic pain and necessitates operative revision, if present. At the present time, radionuclide imaging and subtraction arthrography are effectively utilized in demonstrating loosening as well as other causes of painful total joint prosthesis[20–25] (see Tables 6–2 and 6–3).

### Radionuclide Imaging

Increased activity is normally observed on the radionuclide scan up to six to eight months following surgical implantation. Beyond this period the image should return to normal. Diffuse increased activity and focal increased activity adjacent to the tip of the femoral stem are the most common patterns associated with loosening (Fig. 6–25). More recently, attempts have been made to use the radionuclide scan to distinguish mechanical loosening from infection. On the 99mTc scan, focal increased activity is more consistent with mechanical loosening, while diffuse increased activity should indicate infection.[23, 24] 99mTc and 67Ga imaging (Fig. 6–26) may also help distinguish between the two types of loosening, in that if both scan patterns are incongruent, infection is more likely to be present.[25] Increased activity may normally be observed in the region of the calcar, probably related to increased bone turnover in a high stress region. Radionuclide imaging is also helpful in suggesting causes other than loosening for the patient's pain, such as trochanteric bursitis (Fig. 6–27) or pseudarthrosis in the presence of an osteotomized greater trochanter. Heterotopic bone formation produces increased activity confined to the region of the femoral neck and the adjacent soft tissues, which when observed should suggest this process even though the plain films are normal or equiv-

**Table 6–3.** COMPLICATIONS OF TOTAL HIP PROSTHESES

Dislocation
Loosening
Nonunion or avulsion of greater trochanter
Heterotopic bone
Fractures
Trochanteric bursitis

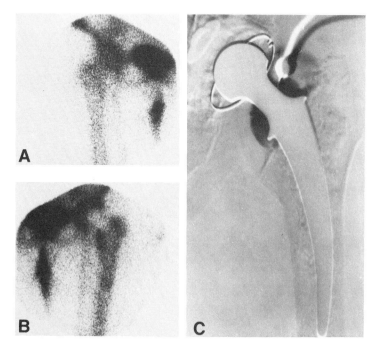

**Figure 6–25.** Diffuse increased activity around the femoral component *(B)* in comparison with the normal opposite side *(A)* indicates loosening, which is confirmed by arthrography *(C)*.

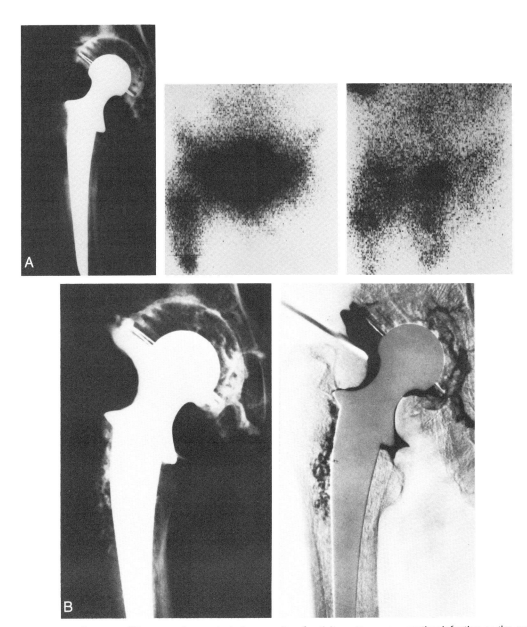

**Figure 6–26.** *A,* $^{99m}$Tc and $^{67}$Ga scans demonstrate incongruity of activity patterns, suggesting infection as the cause of loosening. *B,* Arthrogram confirms loosening of both components and demonstrates fistulous tracts communicating with the acetabular component. Culture of the aspirate grew Staphylococcus. (From Gelman MI, Coleman RE, Stevens PM, Davey BW: Radiography, radionuclide imaging and arthrography in the evaluation of total hip and knee replacement. Radiology *128:*677–682, Sept 1978.)

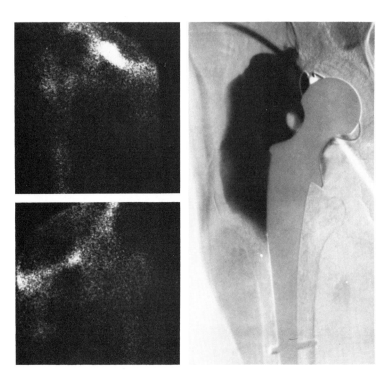

**Figure 6–27.** Trochanteric bursitis. Equivocal radionuclide scan was followed by an arthrogram demonstrating filling of the trochanteric bursa. Characteristic filling of the trochanteric bursa, which is posterior to the greater trochanter, indicates a trochanteric bursitis. (From Gelman MI, Coleman RE, Stevens PM, Davey BW: Radiography, radionuclide imaging and arthrography in the evaluation of total hip and knee replacement. Radiology *128*:677–682, Sept 1978.)

ocal (Fig. 6–28). Frog-leg lateral views will demonstrate increased activity confined to the soft tissues and confirm the diagnosis. If removal of this bone is necessary it must be mature prior to removal or the condition will frequently recur. Although routine radiographs will demonstrate interval maturation of heterotopic bone, the radionuclide scan is a more sensitive modality, demonstrating decreasing activity with maturation.

## Subtraction Arthrography

Subtraction arthrography has been helpful in demonstrating loosening of a prosthesis prior to or in the absence of plain film changes. An anteroposterior roentgenogram of the hip with the foot internally rotated is obtained as is a frog-leg lateral view. Using fluoroscopic image amplification, a metallic marker is placed on the skin over the midpoint of the neck of the femoral component. This point is marked on the skin with indelible ink and the metallic marker is removed. The inguinal ligament as well as the femoral artery should be palpated to make sure the mark is below the ligament and lateral to the artery. The skin is cleansed with povidone-iodine, draped, and locally infiltrated with 1 per cent lidocaine in the

area of the ink mark. A #20 gauge disposable spinal needle is directed straight down onto the metal prosthesis, or obliquely if the pulse is directly over it, under fluoroscopic guidance. Metal-to-metal contact will be felt when the needle point encounters the femoral prosthesis. Having the patient roll into an oblique position will allow observation of the needle point. If fluid is present, as much of it as possible is aspirated. If no fluid can be aspirated, normal saline (without bacteriostatic agent) is injected and aspirated and is then sent to the laboratory for smear, culture, and test for sensitivity of aerobic and anaerobic organisms. Frequently, however, the injected saline cannot be reaspirated. A few drops of Renografin 60 or 76 are injected and, if these flow away from the needle point, the needle is properly positioned. The patient may have to roll into an oblique position in order to observe the contrast material separate from the prosthesis. If the contrast material pools around the needle point, the needle must be repositioned. When the needle is properly positioned, the lower leg and foot are immobilized with sandbags or a head clamp. An anteroposterior roentgenogram is then made with the needle in place. Under fluoroscopic guidance, approximately 15 to 20 ml or more of contrast material is injected through a

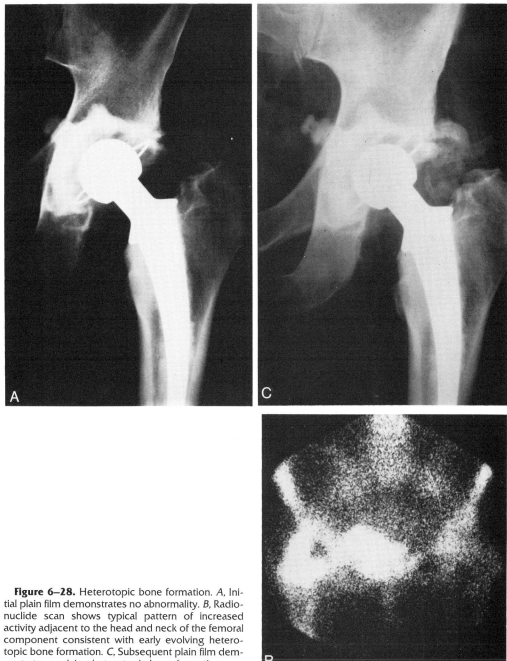

**Figure 6–28.** Heterotopic bone formation. *A,* Initial plain film demonstrates no abnormality. *B,* Radionuclide scan shows typical pattern of increased activity adjacent to the head and neck of the femoral component consistent with early evolving heterotopic bone formation. *C,* Subsequent plain film demonstrates evolving heterotopic bone formation.

connector tube until the capsular space is well filled or the patient complains of a pressure sensation. A second anteroposterior roentgenogram is then taken, making certain the hip remains immobile. These two films are used for the subtraction study. The large volume of contrast material provides adequate filling of the capsular space and ensures seepage of contrast material between the methacrylate and bone or between the prosthesis and the methacrylate if loosening is present, since the subtraction study precludes exercise of the hip before the first two roentgenograms are obtained. The needle is then removed and the hip is exercised passively or actively. Anteroposterior views with and without traction are obtained as are frog-leg and groin lateral views. If motion prevents perfect superimposition of the mask on the radiograph to be subtracted, the study may be salvaged by subtraction of the acetabular and femoral components separately.

**Normal Total Hip Arthrogram.** In the normal total hip arthrogram, contrast medium remains confined by a thick fibrous pseudocapsule, which usually forms within four to five months following surgery. This pseudo-capsule creates a space limited by the rim of the acetabular cup and the base of the neck of the femoral component. Occasionally, contrast medium is noted in the area of the flange or base of the neck of the femoral component but is not associated with loosening. Antegrade and retrograde lymphatic filling, which may normally be observed in the absence of demonstrable infection or loosening, is probably related to a combination of increased pressure during injection and alteration of the lymphatic bed by previous surgery (Fig. 6–29).

**Abnormal Total Hip Arthrogram.** The abnormal total hip arthrogram demonstrates contrast medium beyond the pseudocapsular space. Seepage of contrast material between the methyl methacrylate and bone of either the acetabular or femoral components or between the metal and methyl methacrylate of the femoral component indicates loosening (Fig. 6–30).

Abscess cavities or fistulous tracts may occur with infection (Fig. 6–31). Their demonstration by arthrography is of considerable importance in allowing the orthopedic surgeon to plan the extent of operative exposure and to provide adequate drainage.

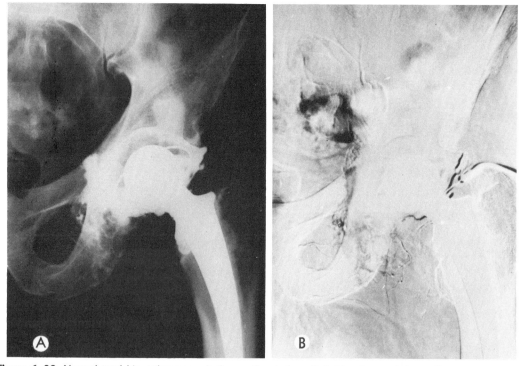

**Figure 6–29.** Normal total hip arthrogram. A, Conventional view. B, Subtraction technique. The contrast medium remains confined to the pseudocapsular space. Lymphatic filling is frequently observed and is normal. (From Gelman MI: Arthrography in total hip prosthesis complications. Am J Roentgenol *126*:743–750, 1976.)

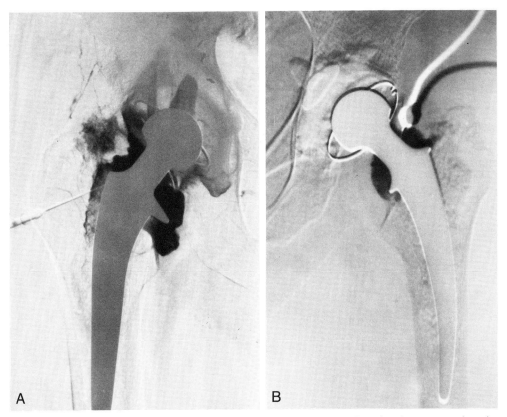

**Figure 6–30.** *A*, Abnormally widened as well as irregular lucent zones at the methacrylate-bone or metal-methacrylate interface constitute plain film evidence of loosening. However, arthrography is required for confirmation. Seepage of contrast medium into the methacrylate-bone interface constitutes arthrographic evidence of loosening. *B*, Contrast media at the metal-methacrylate interface of the femoral component and the polyethylene-methacrylate interface of the acetabular component constitutes arthrographic evidence of acetabular and femoral component loosening.

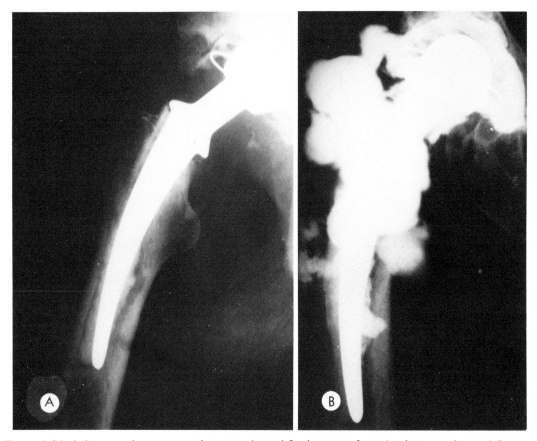

**Figure 6–31.** Arthrogram demonstrates abscess cavity and fistulous tract formation between the medullary canal and the soft tissues of the thigh. (From Gelman MI: Arthrography in total hip prosthesis complications. Am J Roentgenol *126*:743–750, 1976.)

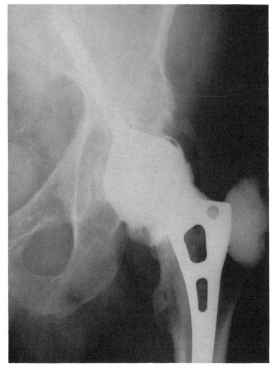

**Figure 6–32.** Trochanteric bursitis, noninfected. Arthrogram demonstrates filling of the trochanteric bursa. Aspirate yielded no growth on culture. (From Gelman MI: Arthrography in total hip prosthesis complications. AJR *126*:743–750, 1976.)

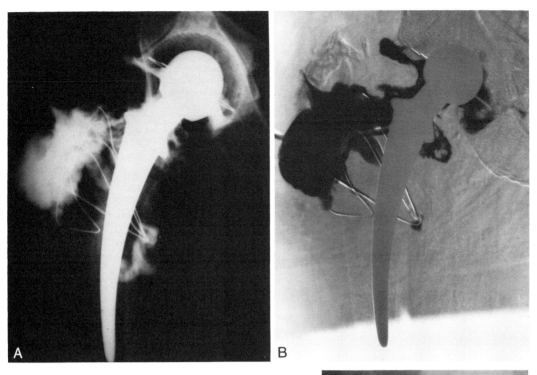

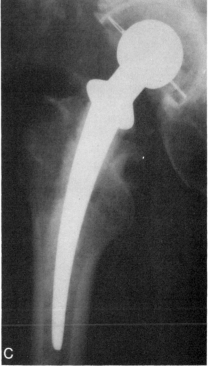

**Figure 6–33.** Trochanteric bursitis, infected. Arthrogram demonstrates filling of the trochanteric bursa as well as fistulous tract formation along the trochanteric osteotomy stabilization wires. Aspirate cultured *Staphylococcus aureus,* coagulose positive. *A,* Arthrogram. *B,* Subtraction technique. *C,* Treatment consisted of excision and drainage of the bursa and fistulous tracts, resection of the greater trochanter and removal of the wires, and antibiotics. The total hip components were not loose.

Although pain in a patient with a total hip prosthesis frequently indicates loosening, arthrography may implicate other causes, necessitating a different type of treatment. Filling of the trochanteric bursa indicates a trochanteric bursitis, which may or may not be infected (Figs. 6–32 and 6–33). Fractures through the greater trochanter may be ununited, or fibrous union may be present. If contrast material is observed in the fracture site on arthrography, nonunion is demonstrated and motion at the fracture site may be the cause of pain (Fig. 6–34). Reapproximation of the fracture fragments with new stabilization wires will promote bony union. More recently, the resurfacing type of total hip prosthesis has been designed, precluding complications associated with the femoral stem (Fig. 6–35A). Loosening, however, may occur with this type of prosthesis as well (Fig. 6–35 B to D).

In summary, routine radiographs may be helpful in determining the presence of a loose total hip prosthesis, but the fact that films are normal does not exclude this possibility. Radionuclide imaging utilizing a $^{99m}$Tc phosphate complex is an effective screening procedure to determine the presence of loosening as well as other complications. If the image is abnormal or equivocal, it should be followed by arthrography. Arthrography will confirm the presence of loosening or demonstrate other possible causes of a positive image, some of which do not require surgical intervention. It also provides fluid for culture and is especially helpful when the radionuclide image results are nonspecific or borderline.

Arthrodesis of the hip involves surgical fusion and is reserved for patients in whom previous surgical procedures have failed or infection has occurred, or in those dependent upon excessive physical activity (e.g., farmers or laborers). It is particularly effective in the young adult or teenager without back, contralateral hip, or knee pain, since increased stress will be placed on these areas (Fig. 6–36).

### Interim or Salvage Procedures

**Colonna Procedure.** The femoral head and entire femoral neck are removed and the greater trochanter is reshaped, covered with capsule or a vitallium cup, and implanted into the acetabulum (Fig. 6–37). This procedure is used mainly in relatively young persons to salvage the hip joint after failure of a prosthesis or after avascular necrosis of the femoral head with subsequent resorption of the femoral neck. In an older patient, total hip replacement would be the procedure of choice.[23]

**Girdlestone Procedure.** The femoral head and neck are removed to salvage the hip following infection or failure of total hip replacement components secondary to infection (Fig. 6–38).[26]

### CONGENITAL DISLOCATION OF THE HIP AND HIP DYSPLASIA

Congenital dislocation of the hip may be treated by a variety of innominate bone os-

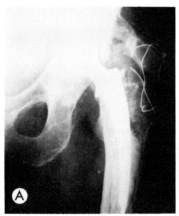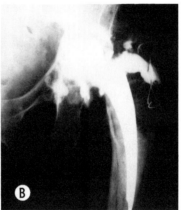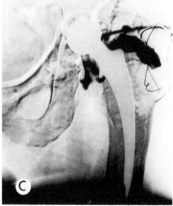

**Figure 6–34.** Arthrogram demonstrating contrast medium in the trochanteric osteotomy site, indicating lack of fibrous union and subsequent pseudarthrosis. A, Plain film. B, Conventional arthrogram. C, Subtraction arthrogram. (From Gelman MI: Arthrography in total hip prosthesis complications. Am J Roentgenol 126:743–750, 1976.)

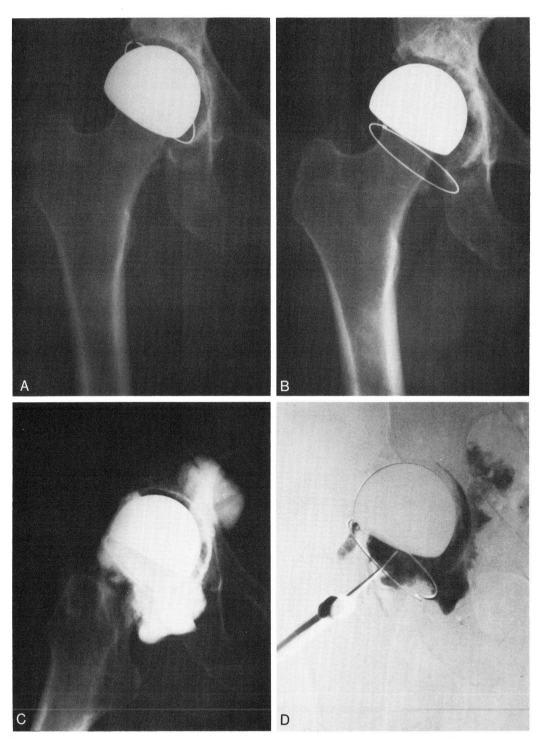

**Figure 6–35.** *A,* Resurfacing type prosthesis. *B* to *D,* Loose acetabular component of resurfacing prosthesis is indicated by displaced ring and confirmed by arthrography.

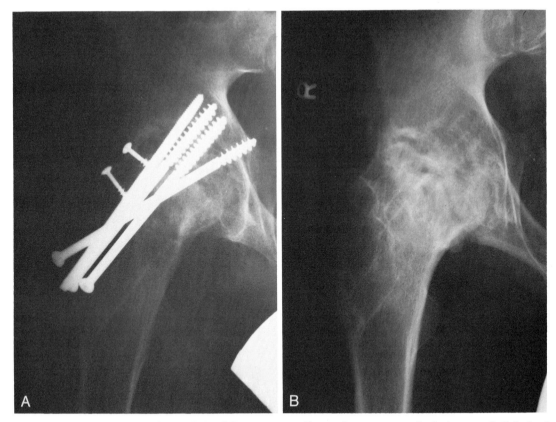

**Figure 6–36.** *A*, Arthrodesis of the right hip following trauma. The smaller screws transfix the bone graft. *B*, Fusion is complete and screws have been removed.

teotomies, the purpose of which is to maintain coverage of the femoral head by realigning the acetabulum.[27] Since concomitant excessive femoral neck anterversion is usually present, correction by a subtrochanteric

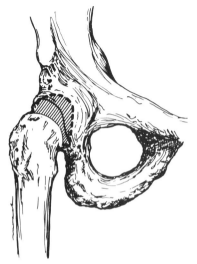

**Figure 6–37.** Colonna procedure.

or supracondylar osteotomy may also be performed (Fig. 6–39).

**Pemberton Osteotomy.** In the Pemberton procedure a curved osteotomy extends from just superior to the anterior inferior iliac spine to the triradiate cartilage. The roof of the acetabulum is rotated anterolaterally with the triradiate cartilage acting as a hinge and a bone graft is placed at the osteotomy site (Fig. 6–40).[28–30]

**Salter Osteotomy.** In the Salter procedure the opening wedge osteotomy extends from the sciatic notch to the anterior inferior iliac spine. The roof of the acetabulum, as well as the pubis and ischium, is rotated anterolaterally, with the symphysis pubis acting as a hinge, and a bone graft is placed at the osteotomy site (Fig. 6–41).[28, 31]

**Chiari Osteotomy.** The Chiari procedure is performed for the irreducible congenitally dislocated hip. It provides a shelf or roof for the femoral head that remains dislocated. The osteotomy line starts lateral and superior to the acetabulum and extends medially at 15 degrees of cephalad angulation. The

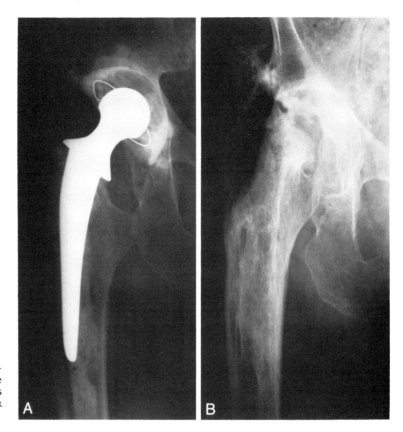

**Figure 6–38.** Girdlestone procedure. *A,* Total hip which became infected. *B,* Total hip components as well as femoral head and neck are removed.

pelvis inferior to the osteotomy is displaced medially, creating a shelf for the subluxed or dislocated femoral head (Fig. 6–42).[27, 32]

**Colonna Capsular Arthroplasty.** This pro-

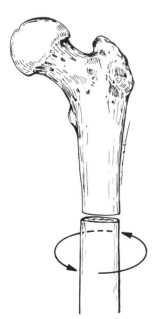

**Figure 6–39.** Supracondylar external rotational osteotomy.

cedure is an arthroplasty that is performed when the acetabulum is underdeveloped, resulting in a newly created, enlarged and deepened acetabular cavity that better accommodates the femoral head.[34]

**Steel Triple Innominate Osteotomy.** This osteotomy incorporates the Salter procedure along with ischial and pubic rami osteotomies. It allows greater rotation of the distal segment in older patients where symphysis pubis mobility is decreased owing to ligamentous rigidity (Fig. 6–43).[33]

**Periacetabular "Dial" Osteotomy.** This osteotomy is curved about the entire circumference of the acetabulum, which is then rotated to provide greater coverage of the femoral head. It is technically difficult and not commonly used, and is effective primarily in adolescents and young adults (Fig. 6–44).[30]

**Femoral Osteotomies.** Femoral osteotomies (proximal or distal) have been utilized in the treatment of many congenital and acquired orthopedic problems. A summary of the indications and various types of osteotomies is seen in Table 6–1.[35]

**Femoral Shortening and Lengthening.** Leg length discrepancy may be treated by epi-

*Text continued on page 130*

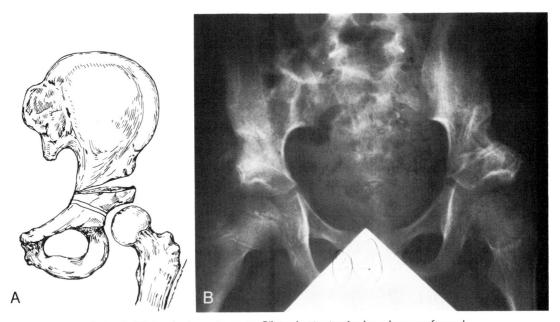

**Figure 6–40.** Pemberton osteotomy. Bilateral osteotomies have been performed.

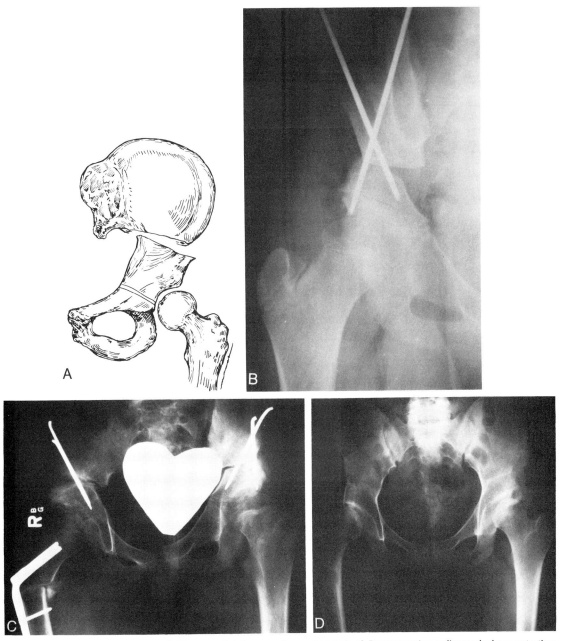

**Figure 6–41.** Salter osteotomy. *A*, Diagram. *B*, Intraoperative radiograph. *C*, Postoperative radiograph demonstrating healing. A proximal femoral osteotomy has also been performed. *D*, Healed osteotomies.

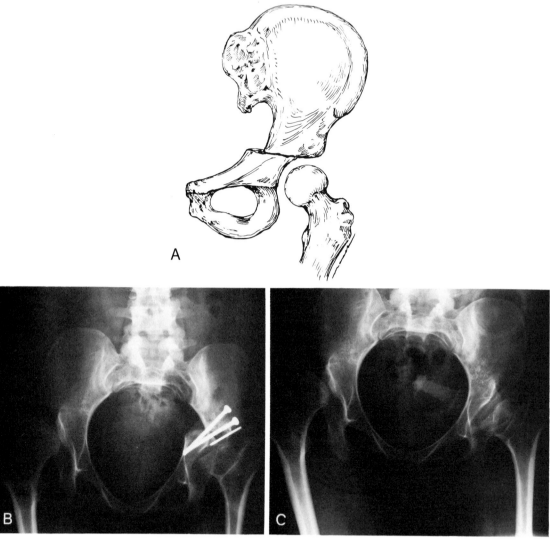

**Figure 6–42.** Chiari osteotomy. *A,* Diagram. *B,* Postoperative radiograph. *C,* Healed osteotomy. Note increased coverage of the left hip postosteotomy as compared with the right.

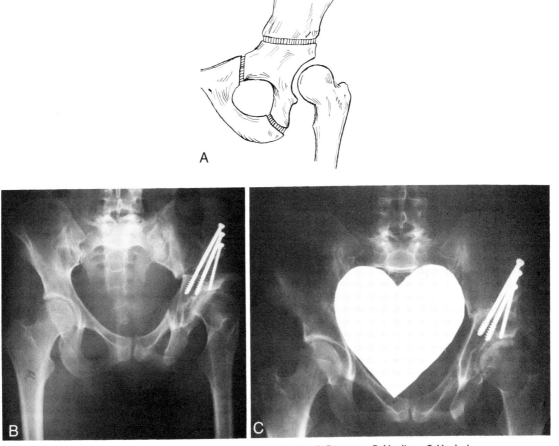

**Figure 6–43.** Steel triple innominate osteotomy. *A*, Diagram. *B*, Healing. *C*, Healed.

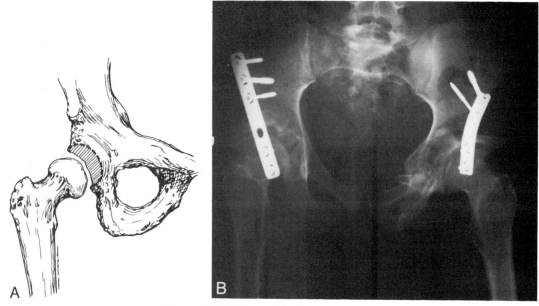

**Figure 6–44.** Periacetabular "dial" osteotomy.

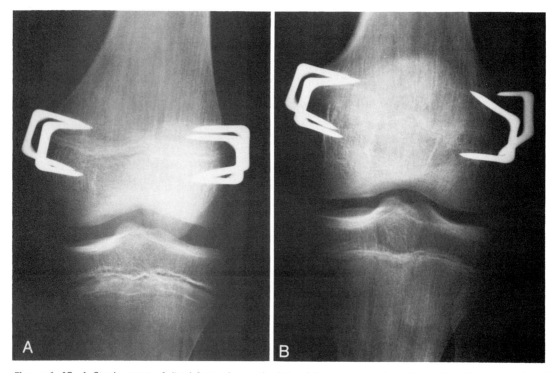

**Figure 6–45.** A, Staple arrest of distal femoral growth plate of the longer leg is performed to alleviate leg length discrepancy. B, Splaying of staples over a three-year period indicates some progressive growth over the interval.

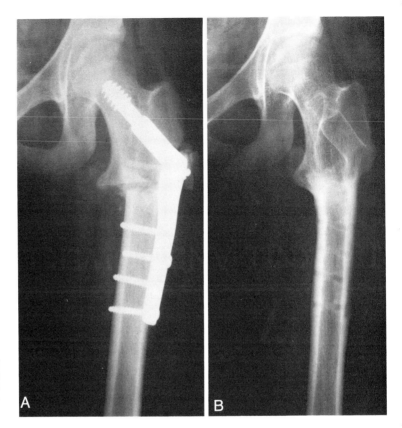

**Figure 6–46.** Femoral shortening accomplished by osteotomy in the subtrochanteric area. *A,* Immediate postosteotomy. *B,* Healed osteotomy.

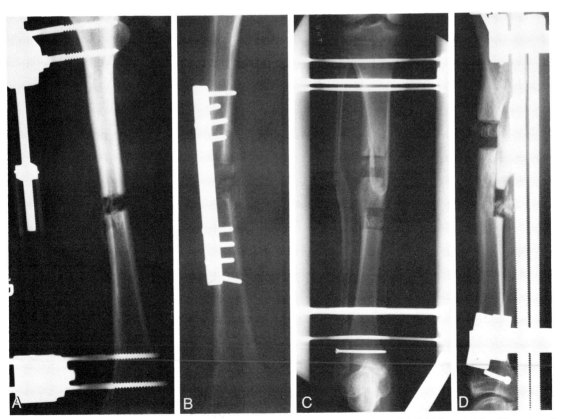

**Figure 6–47.** Femoral lengthening accomplished by a transverse osteotomy. Length is initially maintained by external fixation device *(A),* which is subsequently revised to internal fixation *(B).* A bone graft is in place. *C* and *D,* Femoral lengthening accomplished by a step osteotomy.

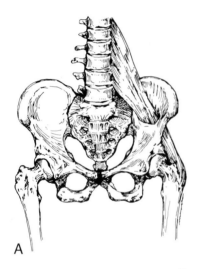
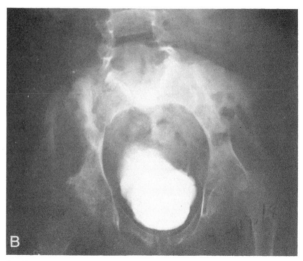

**Figure 6–48.** Mustard procedure.

physiodesis (growth plate arrest) (Fig. 6–45), femoral shortening, or femoral lengthening. Femoral shortening may be accomplished in the subtrochanteric area with metallic fixation of the osteotomized fragments (Fig. 6–46). Femoral lengthening may be achieved by a "Z" or step transverse osteotomy with skeletal traction (Fig. 6–47).[35]

## CORRECTIVE PROCEDURES FOR NEUROMUSCULAR IMBALANCE ABOUT THE HIP

In neuromuscular disease about the hip, abductor and extensor muscle power may be reinforced by transfer of the iliopsoas muscle. This may be accomplished by an anterolateral iliopsoas muscle transfer (Mustard procedure) or a posterior iliopsoas muscle transfer (Sharrard procedure). Clinical features dictate which procedure is utilized. Radiographically, both procedures are characterized by fenestrations in the iliac bone and deformity in the region of or below the greater trochanter, representing the new insertion of the iliopsoas muscle. The defects or fenestrations in the iliac bone are situated more lateral in the anterolateral iliopsoas muscle transfer (Mustard procedure) (Fig. 6–48) than in the posterior iliopsoas muscle transfer (Sharrard procedure) (Fig. 6–49).[36]

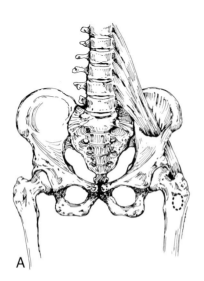
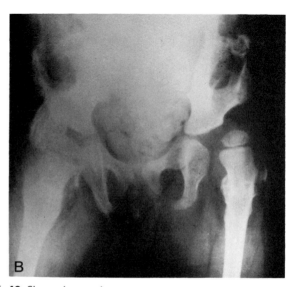

**Figure 6–49.** Sharrard procedure.

# References

1. Massie WK: Treatment of femoral neck fractures emphasizing long term follow-up observations on aseptic necrosis. Clin Orthop 92:16, 1973
2. Bayliss AP, Davidson JK: Traumatic osteonecrosis of the femoral head following intracapsular fracture: incidence and earliest radiological features. Clin Radiol 28:407–414, 1977
3. Asnis SE, Shoji H, Bohne WH: Scintimetric evaluation of complications after femoral neck fractures. Clin Orthop 121:149–156, 1976
4. Outerbridge RE: Perosseous venography in the diagnosis of viability in subcapital fractures of the femur. Clin Orthop 137:132–139, 1978
5. Bonfiglio M, Bardenstein MB: Treatment by bone grafting of aseptic necrosis of the femoral head and nonunion of the femoral neck. J Bone Joint Surg 40A:1329–1346, 1958
6. Bonfiglio M, Voke EM: Aseptic necrosis of the femoral head and nonunion of the femoral neck. J Bone Joint Surg 50A:48–66, 1968
7. Judet R, Judet J, Lord G, Roy-Camille R, Letournel E: Treatment of fractures of the femoral neck by pedicled graft. Presse Med 69:2452–2453, 1961
8. Winter WG, Clawson DK: Complications of treatment of fractures and dislocations of the hip. In Epps CH Jr (ed): Complications in Orthopaedic Surgery J.B. Lippincott Co., Philadelphia 1978, pp. 403–450
9. Coventry MB: Salvage of the painful hip prosthesis. J Bone Joint Surg 46A:200, 1964
10. Whittaker RP, et al.: Fifteen years' experience with metallic endoprosthetic replacement of the femoral head for femoral neck fractures. J Trauma 12:799, 1971
11. Andersson G, Nielsen JM: Results after arthroplasty of the hip with Moore's prosthesis. Acta Orthop Scand 43:397, 1972
12. Dimon JH, Hughston JC: Unstable intertrochanteric fractures of the hip. J Bone Joint Surg 49A:440–450, 1967
13. Naiman PT, Schien AJ, Siffert RS: Medial displacement fixation for severely comminuted intertrochanteric fractures. Clin Orthop 62:151–155, 1969
14. Sarmiento A, Williams EM: The unstable intertrochanteric fracture: treatment with a valgus osteotomy and I-beam nail-plate. J Bone Joint Surg 52A:1309–1318, 1970
15. Naimark A, Kossoff J, Schepsis A: Intertrochanteric fractures: current concepts of an old subject: AJR 133:889–894, 1979
16. Hunter GA, Krajbich IJ: The results of medial displacement osteotomy for unstable intertrochanteric fractures of the femur. Clin Orthop 137:140–143, 1978
17. Mooney V: Fractures of the shaft of the femur. In Rockwood CA, Green DP: Fractures. Vol. 2. J. B. Lippincott Co., Philadelphia, 1975, pp. 1075–1129
18. De Belder KRJ: Distal migration of the femoral intramedullary nail. J Bone Joint Surg 50B:324–333, 1968
19. Baker GI, Rankin EA: Complications of treatment of fractures of the femoral shaft. In Epps CH Jr: Complications in Orthopaedic Surgery. Vol. 1. J. B. Lippincott Co., Philadelphia, 1978, pp. 451–474
20. Gelman MI: Arthrography in total hip prosthesis complications. AJR 126:743–750, 1976
21. DeSmet A, Kramer D, Martel W: The metal-cement interface in total hip prostheses. AJR 129:279–282, 1977
22. Gelman MI, Coleman RE, Stevens PM, Davey BW: Radiography, radionuclide imaging, and arthrography in the evaluation of total hip and knee replacement. Radiology 128:677–682, 1978
23. Weiss PE, Mall JC, Hoffer PB, Munaz WR, Rodrijo JJ, Genant HK: 99mTc-methylene diphosphonate bone imaging in the evaluation of total hip prostheses. Radiology 133:727–729, 1979
24. Williamson, BRJ, McLaughlin RE, Wang G, Miller CW, Teates CD, Bray ST: Radionuclide bone imaging as a means of differentiating loosening and infection in patients with a painful total hip prosthesis. Radiology 133:723–725, 1979
25. Rosenthall L, Lisbona R, Aernandez M, Hadjipavlou A: 99mTc-PP and 67Ga imaging following insertion of orthopedic devices. Radiology 133:717–721, 1979
26. Turek SL: Orthopaedics: Principles and Their Application. 3rd ed. J. B. Lippincott Co., Philadelphia, 1977, pp. 994–1136
27. Gold RH, Amstutz H: Surgical procedures for congenital dislocation of the hip. Radiol Clin N Am 13:123–137, 1975
28. Brinton WR, Lester PD: Hip osteotomies in congenital dislocation of the hip. Appl Radiol 4:49–53, 68, 1975
29. Ryder CT: Congenital dislocation of the hip in the older child: surgical treatment. J Bone Joint Surg 48A:1404–1412, 1966
30. Pemberton PA: Pericapsular osteotomy of the ilium for treatment of congenital subluxation and dislocation of the hip. J Bone Joint Surg 47A:65–86, 1965.
31. Salter RB: Role of innominate osteotomy in the treatment of congenital dislocation and subluxation of the hip in the older child. J Bone Joint Surg 48A:1413–1439, 1966
32. Colton CL: Chiari osteotomy for acetabular dysplasia in young subjects. J Bone Joint Surg 54B:578–589, 1972
33. Coleman SS: Congenital Dysplasia and Dislocation of the Hip. C.V. Mosby Co., St. Louis, 1978, p. 164
34. Colonna PC: Capsular arthroplasty for congenital dislocation of the hip, a two-stage procedure. J Bone Joint Surg 35A:179–197, 1953
35. Ford LT: Osteotomies, nomenclature and uses. Radiol Clin N Am 13:79–92, 1975
36. Ozonoff MB: Orthopedic procedures in neuromuscular disease. Radiol Clin N Am 13:139–156, 1975

# 7

# THE KNEE AND LOWER LEG

## TRAUMA

The knee commonly sustains trauma as a result of industrial, sports, and vehicular accidents. Since it is a diarthrodial weight-bearing joint, significant bony injury requires attention to anatomic restoration in order to avoid debilitating post-traumatic arthritis. Bony injury to the knee may be classified as supracondylar, intercondylar, condylar, patellar, or proximal-tibial in location. Treatment may be closed or open, with rigid internal fixation, depending upon the ease and maintenance of reduction as well as the experience of the orthopedic surgeon[1] (Figs. 7–1 and 7–2). The supracondylar region extends from the femoral condyles to the junction of the metaphysis with the femoral shaft. When displacement is present, it is usually posterior and associated with posterior angulation owing to the hamstring and gastrocnemius muscle pull (Fig. 7–3). A fat-blood level in the suprapatellar bursa indicates that a fracture has an intra-articular component and the fat and blood from the marrow cavity have seeped into the joint and communicating bursa (Fig. 7–4A). Patellar fractures are most commonly transverse in type, secondary to an indirect force provided by hypercontraction of the quadriceps and patellar tendons such as occurs with acute flexion of the knee. A direct force usually results in a comminuted fracture (Fig. 7–4B). If patellar fracture fragment separation is excessive, wire fixation in the form of tension band or cerclage wire may be utilized (Fig. 7–5). Total patellectomy is recommended in comminuted fractures where no large fragment remains.

Tibial condylar fractures, if sufficiently depressed, require open reduction and fixation to prevent subsequent abnormal axial alignment and abnormal unicompartmental stress resulting in post-traumatic degenerative arthritis. Depressed condylar fractures may be operatively elevated and reinforced with bone graft from the iliac crest (Fig. 7–6) or with metallic fixation (transverse bolt, AO cancellous screws, buttress plate and screws).[1,2] Tomography may help in confirming the extent of the fracture and in delineating the anteroposterior intracapsular location of the larger fragments, aiding the orthopedic surgeon in his operative approach.[3,4]

Varus or valgus stress films under general or spinal anesthesia are helpful in demonstrating ligamentous injury, commonly associated with certain fractures such as depressed lateral tibial condylar fractures. Widening of the medial or lateral joint compartment with valgus or varus stress greater than 1 cm is highly suggestive of collateral ligament instability.[5] Occasionally, this may be appreciated on the initial nonstress films (Fig. 7–7). The presence of a staple horizontally oriented to the knee joint indicates a previous collateral ligament repair (Fig. 7–8).

Fractures of the intercondylar eminence or tibial spine indicate probable associated cruciate ligament injury. The cruciate ligaments may be demonstrated by arthrography, but computed tomography has also been utilized recently (Fig. 7–9).[6,7] Bowing of the anterior cruciate ligament with an anterior drawer maneuver indicates a lax ligament or incomplete tear. Nonvisualiza-

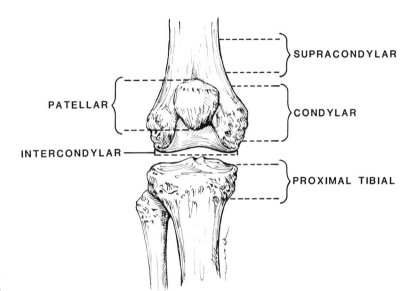

**Figure 7–1.** Anatomic classification of bony injuries of the knee.

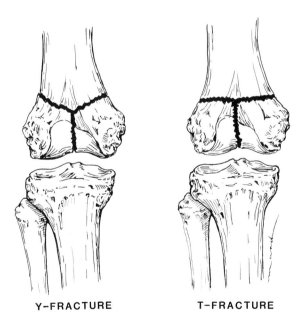

Y-FRACTURE          T-FRACTURE

**Figure 7–2.** Combined supracondylar and intercondylar fractures of the distal femur may be classified as Y or T fractures.

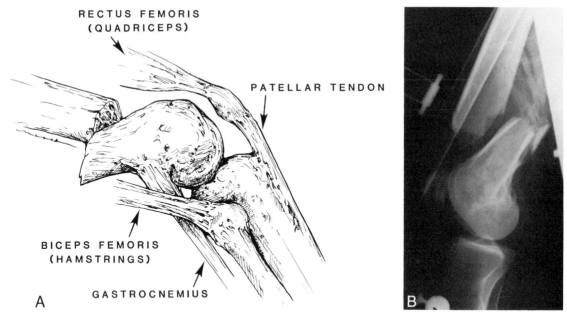

**Figure 7–3.** Supracondylar fracture with posterior displacement and angulation.

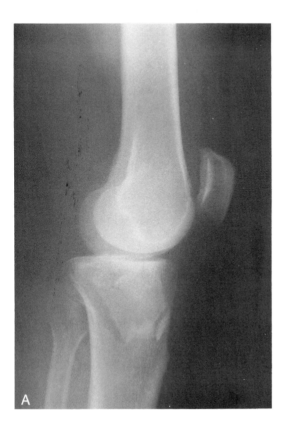

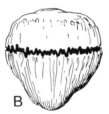
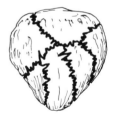

**Figure 7–4.** *A*, Fat-blood level indicating intra-articular fracture. *B*, Transverse and comminuted fractures of the patella.

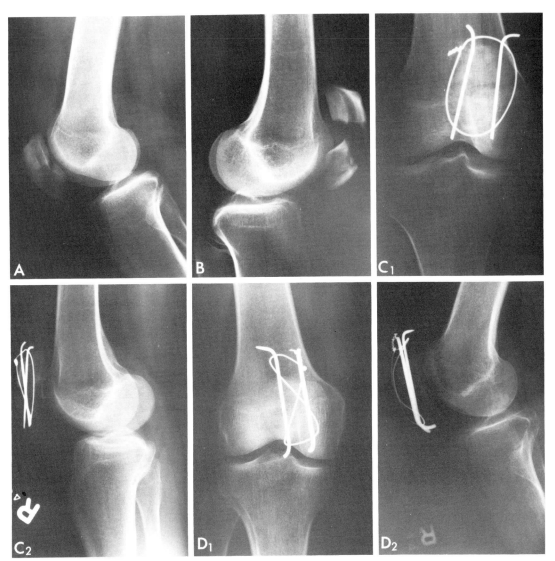

**Figure 7–5.** Nondistracted *(A)* and distracted *(B)* fractures of the patella due to hypercontraction of the quadriceps tendon and patellar ligament. *C* and *D,* Pin and wire internal fixation is utilized in the treatment of patellar fractures.

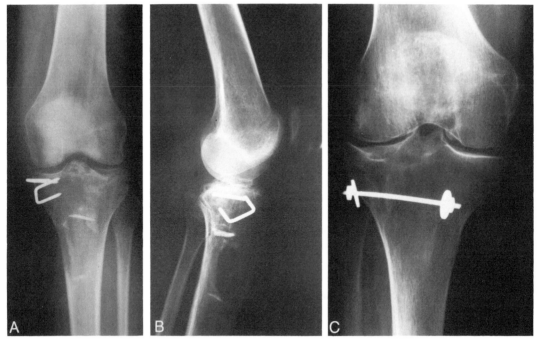

**Figure 7–6.** Depressed condylar fractures of the tibia may be elevated by bone graft *(A and B)* (note fenestration through which bone graft is pushed to elevate fracture) or metallic fixation *(C)*.

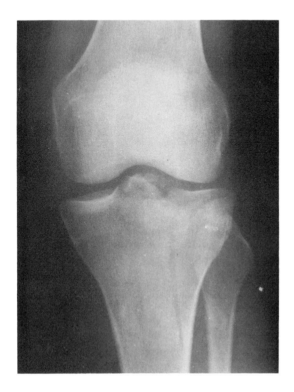

**Figure 7–7.** Lateral tibial condyle fractures are frequently associated with medial collateral ligament instability. When this is not appreciated on routine films, stress views under local or general anesthesia are useful. Note widening of the medial joint compartment with valgus stress, indicating medial collateral ligament laxity.

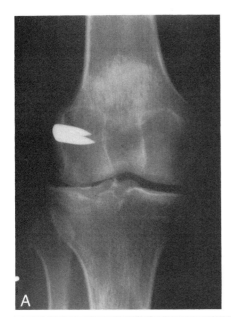

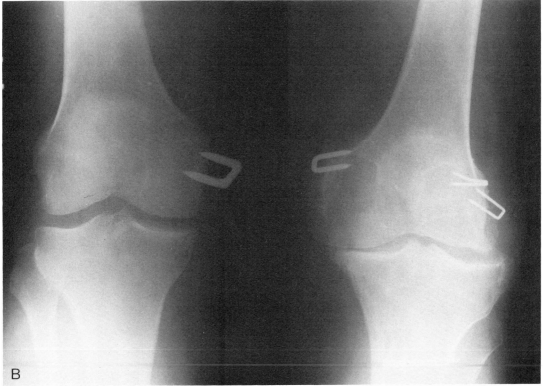

**Figure 7–8.** *A,* Previous lateral collateral ligament repair. *B,* Previous medial and lateral collateral ligament repair with subsequent loosening of staples.

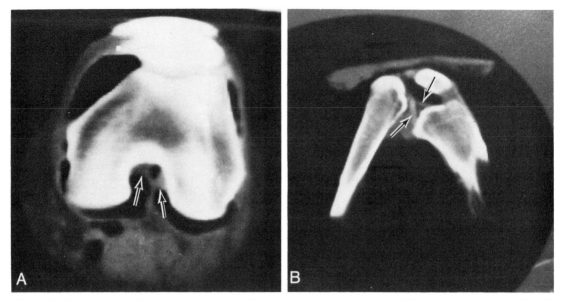

**Figure 7–9.** Computerized tomogram of cruciate ligaments (arrows) requires prior injection of contrast medium for visualization. *A,* Knee of a patient following a double contrast arthrogram. *B,* Knee of a cadaver following instillation of air.

tion of the anterior cruciate ligament with an anterior drawer maneuver may indicate that the ligament is torn (Fig. 7–10); however, tomography may be required to be absolutely certain.[8] At times, complete avulsion of the anterior cruciate ligament from its femoral attachment may be diagnosed by observing an elliptical density in the region of the intercondylar eminence on the arthrogram (Fig. 7–11). This density, coated with positive contrast medium and outlined by air, represents the retracted torn anterior cruciate ligament.[9] This observation would argue utilizing a fluoroscopic field wide enough to include the meniscus as well as the intercondylar eminence of the tibia. Care must be taken not to confuse the ligamentum mucosum, a synovial reflection anterior to

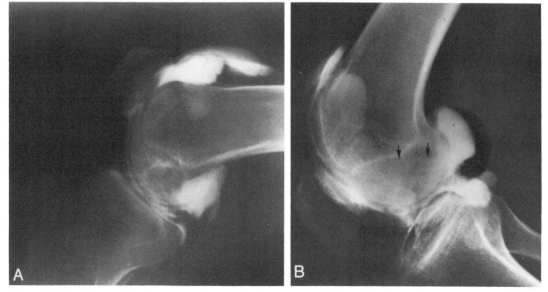

**Figure 7–10.** *A,* Incomplete tear of anterior cruciate ligament, as indicated by sigmoid-shaped configuration with anterior drawer maneuver. *B,* Complete tear of anterior cruciate ligament, as indicated by nonvisualization of the anterior cruciate ligament and good visualization of the posterior cruciate ligament (arrows).

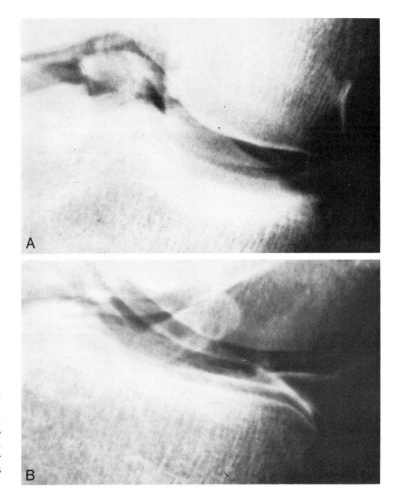

**Figure 7–11.** *A* and *B*, Complete avulsion of the anterior cruciate ligament. Elliptical density in intercondylar eminence region coated by positive contrast medium and outlined by air represents the anterior cruciate ligament avulsed from its femoral attachment.

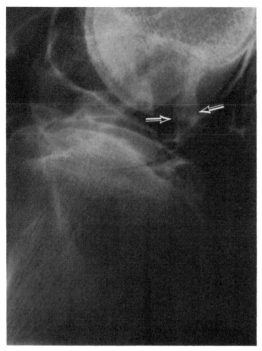

**Figure 7–12.** Ligamentum mucosum (arrows) is a synovial reflection anterior to the anterior cruciate ligament and should not be confused for it.

the anterior cruciate ligament, with the anterior cruciate ligament (Fig. 7–12).

### Tibial Shaft Fractures

Healing of tibial shaft fractures is most dependent upon the extent of initial displacement, comminution, and soft tissue injury, since these factors may directly affect compromise of blood supply.[10] The greater the degree of displacement, comminution, or soft tissue injury, the greater the chance of delayed union or nonunion. Although controversy exists concerning the most significant blood supply to the tibia, the metaphyseal intramedullary blood supply is felt to be the most important, with the periosteal blood supply assuming a more secondary role.[11] Knee and ankle joint surfaces should be parallel to avoid abnormal distribution of weight to these joints; therefore close attention to angulation and rotation is required, even though greater amounts of displacement are allowed. Up to 5 to 10 degrees of angulation in the anteroposterior or lateral plane is considered acceptable. Significant shortening or distraction is to be avoided to

prevent subsequent leg length discrepancy or delayed union or nonunion.[12]

**Treatment.** Recently, closed reduction has been utilized more commonly employing a patellar-tendon-bearing (PTB) below-the-knee cast with cast wedging if the position is unsatisfactory. This allows early weight bearing with decreased joint stiffness and muscle wasting.[13] Steinmann pins on both sides of the fracture site and incorporated into a plaster cast may also be utilized as can traction (Fig. 7–13). The proper site of pin insertion is 1 inch posterior to and 1 inch distal to the tibial tubercle.[14] Compression plating or intramedullary nailing with a Lottes or Kuntscher nail may be used when closed reduction is not realistic or practical (Fig. 7–14). Pins above and below the fracture site in association with a Roger-Anderson external fixation device may be utilized when an open wound or soft tissue loss is present (Fig. 7–15).

When traction is utilized, portable films are obtained and checked for proper position of fracture fragments and to ensure distrac-

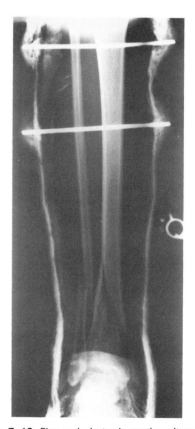

**Figure 7–13.** Pins-and-plaster is another alternative in the treatment of tibial fractures.

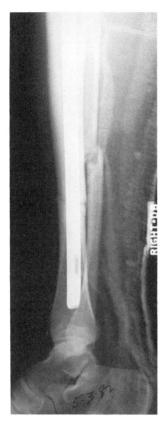

**Figure 7–14.** Lottes or Kuntscher intramedullary nail fixation of tibial fracture.

tion is not present. A gap of more than 0.5 cm delays the healing time to 12 to 18 months, and a gap greater than 1 cm will require 18 to 24 months for healing.[12, 15]

### Radiographic Manifestations of Complications

The more common complications of tibial shaft fractures that may be evident and evaluated radiographically include delayed union, nonunion, malunion, shortening, infection, and vascular injury (Fig. 7–16). Delayed union of a tibial fracture is regarded as lack of bony union after 20 weeks and is diagnosed on the basis of time elapsed and radiographic evidence of little callus formation.[10]

Many factors may cause delayed or nonunion; however, the use of pin fixation through a plaster cast for stabilization may cause persistent distraction that is evident radiographically and may account for delayed union or nonunion.[14] In the presence of infection, drainage at the fracture site may or may not be present.[16] If it is present, sinography will help to delineate the extent of the sinus in the soft tissues as well as whether or not it communicates with the bone. Anteroposterior and lateral films are used to obtain this information, as well as oblique views (Fig. 7–17). Resorption of bone at the fracture site as well as periosteal reaction extending away from the fracture site radiographically suggest an infected nonunion. A radionuclide scan demonstrating increased activity extending a distance from the fracture site is also suggestive of complicating osteomyelitis. A ring sequestrum is an area of radiolucency surrounding a pin tract resulting from infection. If drainage at the pin site or other signs of inflammation are present, treatment includes pin removal, excision of the sequestrum, and antibiotic therapy. Ring sequestra usually heal with time, but until healing has occurred they serve as areas of weakness that may allow further fracture to occur.[14]

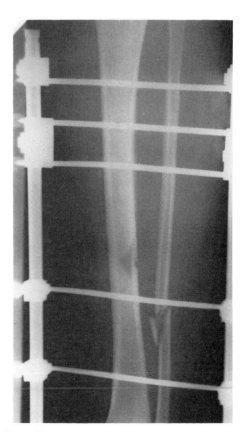

**Figure 7–15.** External fixation device is utilized when open wound, soft tissue loss, or burns are present. The skin is disrupted at the site of the tibial and fibular fractures, necessitating external fixation.

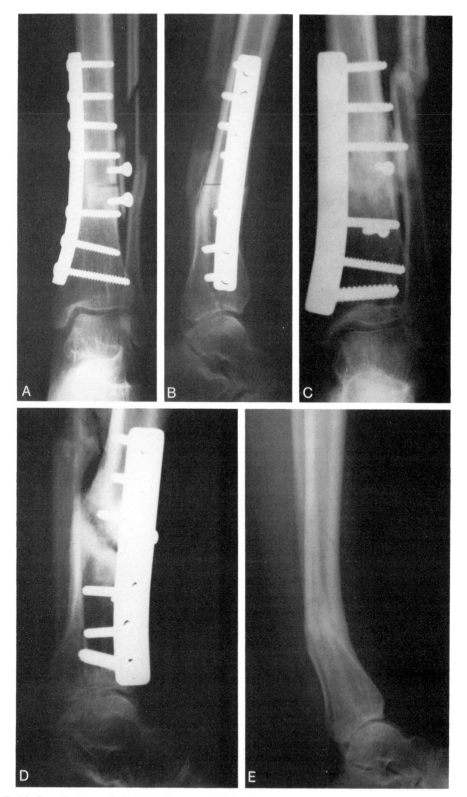

**Figure 7–16.** Complications of tibial shaft fractures include: *A* and *B*, Delayed union necessitating bone graft. *C* and *D*, Nonunion. *E*, Malunion.

and stimulate healing. Inadequate fibular resection and removal of the periosteum will allow regeneration of the fibula and persistent distraction at the tibial fracture site.[15, 18]

Bone graft may be directly applied to the fracture site without associated internal fixation.[12]

When extensive bone loss is present in the tibia, the fibula may be utilized by inducing union between the tibia and fibula and the interosseous membrane or by peg grafting the fibula to the tibia on either side of the area of tibial bone loss (Fig. 7–18).[19-22]

### Fibular Shaft Fractures

Fibular shaft fractures usually accompany tibial shaft fractures and indicate absorption of significant force. Treatment is the same for both; however, the fibula is not involved in weight bearing and functions as a source of muscle and interosseous membrane insertion. Proximal fibular shaft fractures may be associated with posterior malleolar fractures (Maissoneuf fracture) and, therefore, a lateral view of the ankle should be obtained (Fig. 7–19).

### Tibial Plafond Fractures

Fractures of the superior articular surface of the distal tibia or the tibial plafond are important because they involve the articular surface of a weight-bearing joint. Since the posterior tibial margin is important in preventing posterior subluxation of the talus, if the fracture involves 25 per cent or more of the posterior tibial surface, the ankle is rendered unstable, and open reduction and internal fixation are usually carried out (Fig. 7–20).[23]

### Meniscal Injuries

Injuries to the meniscus may occur following trauma and are readily demonstrated by arthrography. Limited excision of the torn portion of the meniscus is the current practice, since removal of the entire meniscus obviates its effect as a shock absorber, resulting in accelerated unicompartmental degenerative arthritis. Complete excision of the meniscus may be recognized radiographi-

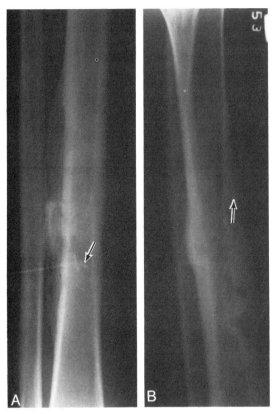

**Figure 7–17.** Anteroposterior and lateral views *(A and B)* of sinogram demonstrate communication of the sinus with the underlying bone (arrows).

Vascular injury resulting from tibial shaft fractures is rare. When it does occur, the anterior tibial artery is most commonly involved, necessitating arteriography. Anterior compartment syndrome follows less significant tibial fractures in which the interosseous membrane is not disrupted and consists of increased pressure within the anterior tibial compartment, which is bounded by the tibia, the fascia of the anterior compartment, the fibula, and the interosseous membrane. Increased pressure caused by hemorrhage and edema lead to occlusion of the anterior tibial artery, resulting in pain over the anterior tibial compartment muscles and sensory deficit in the toes. Treatment consists of emergency fasciotomy.[17]

### Radiographic Manifestations of Treatment of Nonunion

The fibula may be resected to allow compression of the tibial fracture fragments

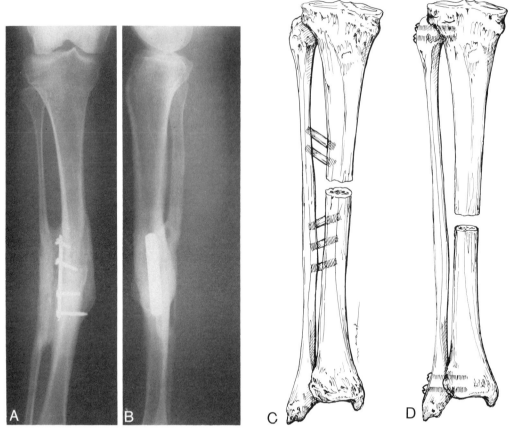

**Figure 7–18.** *A* and *B,* Tibiofibular synostosis to induce healing of a tibial nonunion. *C,* Crosspeg-grafting. *D,* Double tibiofibular synostosis.

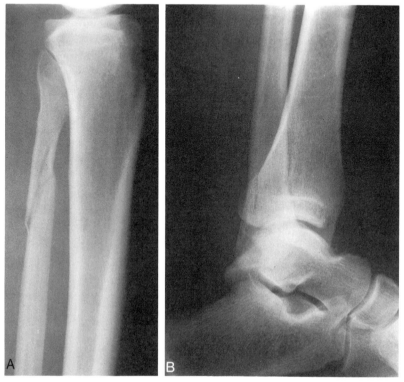

**Figure 7–19.** *A* and *B,* Maissoneuf fracture. Fracture of posterior tibial malleolus in association with a proximal fibular fracture.

144

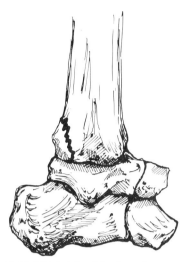

**Figure 7–20.** Tibial plafond fracture. Assessment of the posterior tibial surface is important in determining instability of the ankle, since greater than 25 per cent involvement renders the ankle unstable.

cally, as early as five months postoperatively, by flattening of the femoral condyle (Fig. 7–21), squaring of the tibial condyle, sclerosis of the tibial plateau, and narrowing of the affected joint compartment.[24-27] Osteochondritis dissecans is a focal area of avascular necrosis, usually in the medial femoral

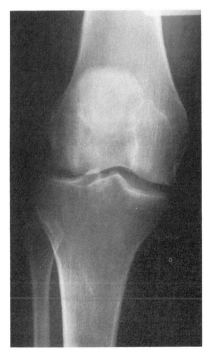

**Figure 7–21.** Early bony changes following complete meniscectomy include flattening of the medial femoral condyle.

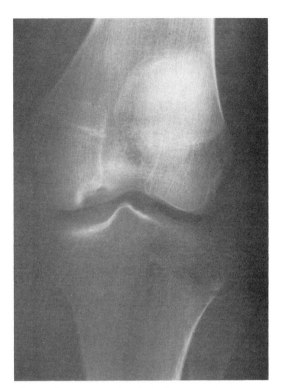

**Figure 7–22.** Osteochondritis dissecans is indicated by a scooped-out defect in the medial femoral condyle.

condyle, involving the subchondral bone (Fig. 7–22). Arthrography is necessary to determine whether the overlying cartilage is disrupted.[28]

**Osteochondral Fractures**

Osteochondral fractures may occur off of the lateral femoral condyle or medial surface of the patella owing to dislocation or relocation of the patella, or off of the medial femoral condyle caused by torsional force on the weight-bearing knee or a direct anterior blow to the patella in a flexed knee (Fig. 7–23). In the majority of cases, the fragments contain both bone and cartilage, and hence routine radiographs of the knee are often diagnostic.[29]

**Chondral Fractures**

Intra-articular fractures may occur in the weight-bearing portion of the distal femur in the uncalcified cartilage, the calcified cartilage, or the subchondral bone. In adolescents these fractures are usually seen in the sub-

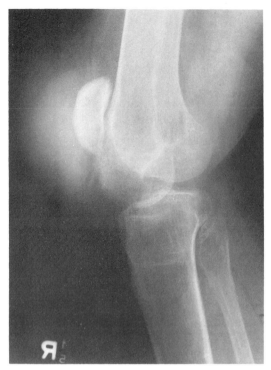

**Figure 7–23.** An osteochondral fracture of the anterior surface of the femoral condyle (scooped-out defect) is noted in association with a large prepatellar hematoma.

chondral bone due to the lack of calcified cartilage and the elasticity of the articular cartilage, but in adults they often occur at the junction of the calcified and uncalcified cartilage, the so-called "tide mark."[29] Depending on where the fracture occurs, the result may be an osteochondral or pure chondral fragment. In osteochondral fractures, separate radiodense fragments are almost always identified on routine radiographs of the knee, whereas chondral fractures require additional diagnostic procedures for delineation and specific diagnosis. Although chondral fractures are observed by the orthopedic surgeon during arthroscopy, they have not been fully appreciated by the radiologist on arthrography, probably because the articular cartilage has largely been ignored and the fluoroscopic field has been kept small.

Chondral fractures of the knee represent one of the "meniscal mimics" in orthopedic practice, since the clinical history and symptoms are very similar to those of a torn meniscus. In fact, chondral fractures may frequently be accompanied by a meniscal tear. In addition, there is often a rapid (less than 24 hours) onset of a hemarthrosis.

The medial femoral condyle is the most common site of involvement, with fractures resulting from a twisting or torque-like force applied to the weight-bearing knee or from direct trauma to the patella. We postulate that during a pivotal injury the anterior tibial spine rotates into the condyle, resulting in a fracture of the medial femoral condyle. Because of the forces involved, there is often an associated tear or partial tear of the anterior cruciate ligament. In the direct blow type of fracture, the undersurface of the patella strikes the medial femoral condyle, resulting in a stellate-appearing fracture. This is exemplified in the dashboard type injury to the knee. In each of our cases, the plain films of the knee were nondiagnostic, and a preoperative diagnosis of chondral fracture was made by arthrography and arthroscopy.[30]

During routine arthrography the field size should be large enough to include both the meniscus and the intercondylar notch region in order to visualize the entire articular surface. We have also occasionally found chondral fractures or fragments on the side opposite that being examined. Initially, only minimal irregularity in the articular surface may be noted, but with careful positioning, a fracture line or fragment will be identified. Two separate patterns are seen. The most common is that of a linear fracture through the articular cartilage with an adjacent cartilage fragment. However, only a scooped-out defect in the condyle may be noted without an associated donor site fragment seen (Fig. 7–24). Because of the difficulty in identifying the chondral fracture using arthrography, arthroscopy is recommended if the arthrogram is negative or equivocal and the patient has persistent symptoms following a knee injury.

Therapeutically, the chondral fracture may be curetted followed by drilling into the subchondral bone to stimulate fibrocartilage healing. This can be done either through the arthroscope or by surgery. Follow-up reveals that less than 50 per cent of these knees will return to normal function.[30]

## ARTHRITIS

Surgery for arthritis of the knee involves osteotomy, arthroplasty, or arthrodesis.

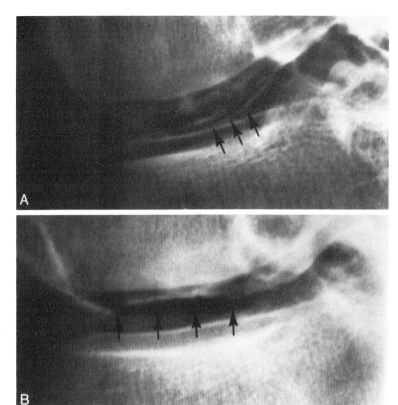

**Figure 7–24.** Chondral fractures demonstrated by arthrography. *A,* There is a linear fracture through the articular cartilage with an adjacent cartilage fragment (arrows). Note the presence of air between the subchondral bone and chondral fragment. *B,* There is a scooped-out defect in the articular cartilage.

Osteotomy is effectively utilized in the treatment of unicompartmental degenerative arthritis of the knee with an associated varus or valgus deformity. Moderate to severe valgus deformity is corrected by distal femoral osteotomy, whereas varus and mild valgus deformities are corrected by proximal tibial osteotomy. Osteotomy is contraindicated in the presence of bicompartmental disease or ligamentous instability. Weight-bearing radiographic views are helpful in determining the actual extent of compartmental narrowing. When excessive varus or valgus deformity is present, stress views of the knee are helpful in evaluating accurately the cartilage in the opposite compartment (Fig. 7–25).

The amount of angular deformity of the knee is determined from a standing anteroposterior view. The angle of the wedge of bone to be removed is determined by adding 5 mm for normal valgus and 5 mm for overcorrection to the amount of existing angular deformity (each degree of angulation being equivalent to 1 mm of bone at the base of the wedge removed). Therefore, if the radiograph shows 5 degrees of varus deform-

ity, a wedge of bone 15 mm thick at the base is removed. The upper cut of the osteotomy parallels and is 2 cm below the articular surface of the proximal tibia, and both cuts are proximal to the tibial tubercle. The fibular head is excised to provide better surgical exposure and lessen the chances of medial displacement of the distal tibial segment. The staple, if utilized, maintains fixation and compression at the osteotomy site (Fig. 7–26). The opening wedge is placed laterally to correct varus deformity and medially to correct mild valgus deformity. If the valgus deformity is moderate to severe, a distal femoral osteotomy is preferentially performed. Operative films demonstrate Kirschner guidewires used to localize the site of the osteotomy (Fig. 7–27). Postoperative radiographic evaluation of the proximal tibial osteotomy should include assessment for healing of the osteotomy, alignment of the osteotomized segments (Fig. 7–28), and recurrence of varus deformity. Delayed union is rare, and nonunion has not been reported.[31, 32] Infection may occur as a complication, but noncasted films are required for adequate evaluation (Fig. 7–29). The pre-

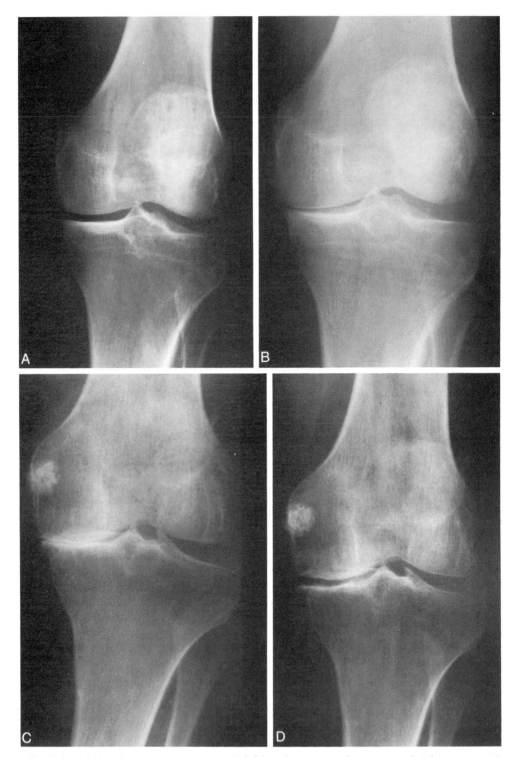

**Figure 7–25.** Weight-bearing or stress views are helpful in determining the amount of deformity as well as the integrity of the articular cartilage in the opposite compartment. Supine and weight-bearing views demonstrate the extent of varus deformity. The supine view (A) demonstrates minimal narrowing of medial joint compartment whereas weight-bearing view (B) demonstrates marked narrowing, indicating extensive cartilage loss. Weight-bearing view (C) indicates marked cartilage loss in the medial joint compartment. Because of associated varus deformity, a valgus stress view (D) is performed to evaluate cartilage in the lateral joint compartment, which is maintained.

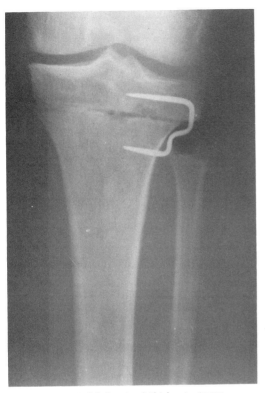

**Figure 7–26.** Proximal tibial osteotomy.

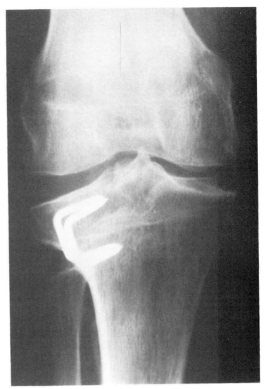

**Figure 7–28.** Healed proximal tibial osteotomy.

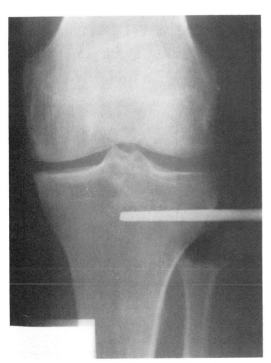

**Figure 7–27.** Operative film with guide.

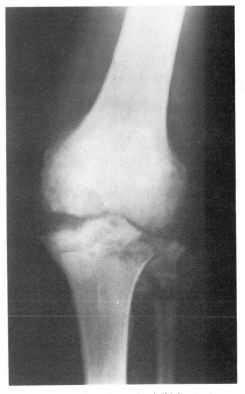

**Figure 7–29.** Infected proximal tibial osteotomy.

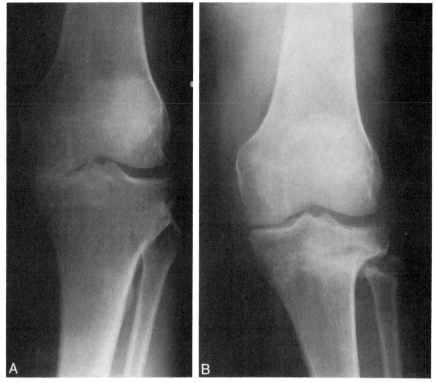

**Figure 7–30.** Preproximal *(A)* and postproximal *(B)* tibial osteotomy weight-bearing radiographs demonstrate medial compartmental widening postoperatively.

viously narrowed compartment may or may not show widening postoperatively, and reformation of articular cartilage following osteotomy has been shown to occur (Fig. 7–30).[33]

**Total Knee Arthroplasty**

Total knee replacement is utilized primarily in the treatment of osteoarthritis, rheumatoid arthritis, and post-traumatic arthritis of the knee. The two main types of total knee prostheses utilized are the hinge unit and the resurfacing unit (Fig. 7–31), which are designed to treat bicompartmental disease (Table 7–1). Occasionally, the resurfacing prosthesis is used to replace only one

**Table 7–1.** TOTAL KNEE PROSTHESES

| | |
|---|---|
| Pin-hinge: | Walldius |
| | Shiers |
| | Guepar |
| Resurfacing: | Polycentric |
| | Geometric |
| | Freeman-Swanson |
| | Duo-patellar |

side of the tibiofemoral joint. The hinge unit is reserved for patients with marked instability due to ligamentous laxity, such as results from rheumatoid arthritis. In this case, the function of the ligaments is replaced by the metal hinge. The rigidity of this prosthesis, however, facilitates loosening or fracturing of the underlying bone. The resurfacing prosthesis consists of a metal femoral component and a polyethylene tibial component, which are cemented in place with methyl methacrylate. Occasionally, screws may be placed into the femoral condyles when insufficient bone is present in order to provide support for the methyl methacrylate (Fig. 7–32). Patellar realignment may also be performed at the same time as total knee arthroplasty (Fig. 7–33).

Postoperatively, plain films are obtained to check for positioning of the tibial component as well as for axial alignment of the knee. The tibial component should be implanted perpendicular to the tibial shaft, since tilting will increase stress at the bone-cement interface, contributing to loosening (Fig. 7–34).[34] Excessive varus or valgus alignment with weight bearing may also facilitate

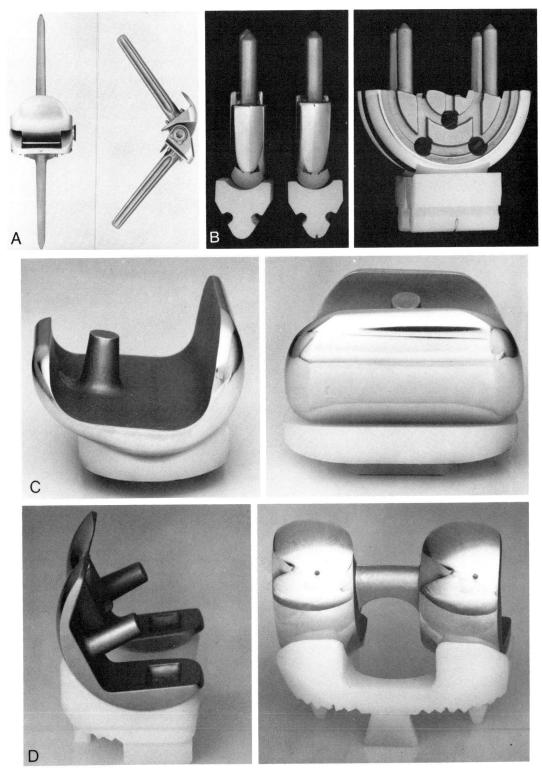

**Figure 7–31.** Two main types of total knee prostheses: *A*, Pin-hinge unit. Types of resurfacing units include: *B*, Polycentric. *C*, Freeman-Swanson. *D*, Geometric.

*Illustration continued on following page*

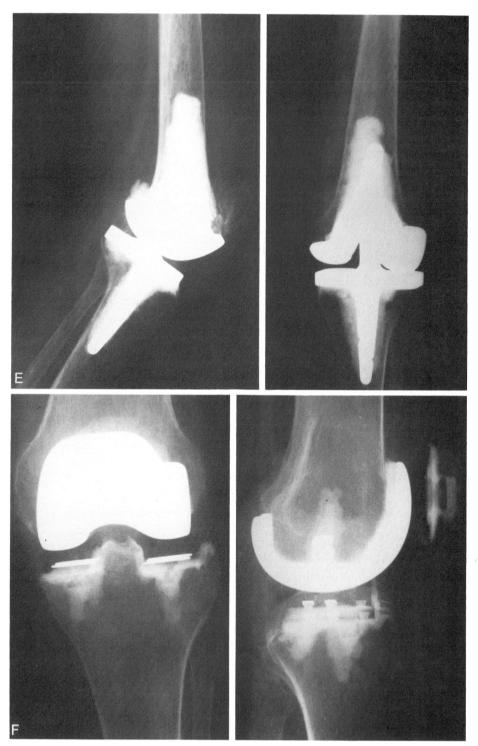

**Figure 7–31.** *Continued E,* Spherocentric. *F,* Duopatellar (note patellar prosthesis). (From Gelman MI, Dunn HK: The radiology of knee joint replacement. AJR *27*:447–455, 1976.)

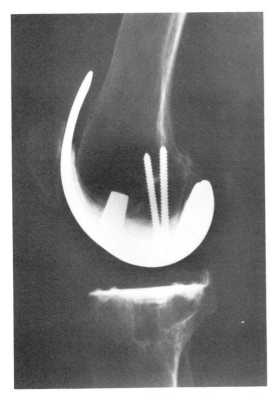

**Figure 7–32.** Screws provide increased support for methylmethacrylate when underlying bone loss is significant.

loosening. A lucent zone between the methyl methacrylate affixing the tibial component and the underlying bone may normally develop early. It should not be greater than 1 to 2 mm in width and should be smooth in contour.

### Technique for Arthrography of Total Knee Prosthesis

The patient is supine and the lower leg immobilized with sandbags or a clamp. If the patella has not been removed, the needle is advanced under the patella into the patellofemoral joint space in the same manner that a conventional arthrogram is performed. If the patella has been removed, the joint space between the femoral and tibial components is marked laterally on the skin with a felt-tip pen under fluoroscopic guidance. The skin is prepared and draped, and the lateral aspect is locally infiltrated with 1 per cent lidocaine. A #20 gauge needle is advanced into the lateral aspect of the knee joint space, and the position is checked fluoroscopically. A tiny amount of contrast medium is injected and, if flow away from

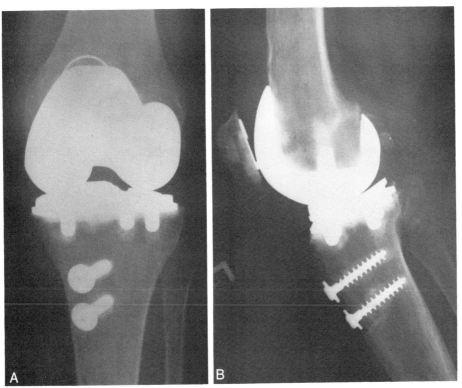

**Figure 7–33.** Patellar realignment (screws in proximal tibia) has been performed in addition to total knee arthroplasty.

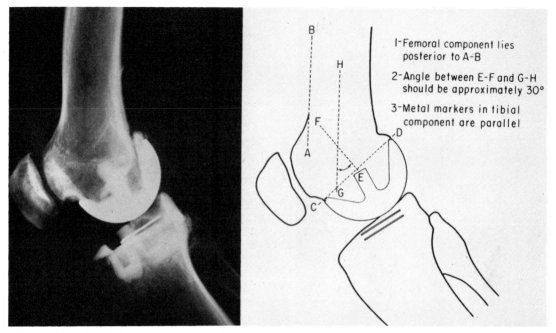

**Figure 7–34.** The tibial component should be perpendicular to the tibial shaft since tilting will concentrate stress, facilitating loosening at the methacrylate-bone interface. (From Gelman MI, Dunn HK: The radiology of knee joint replacement. AJR 27:447–455, 1976.)

the needle is observed, the intra-articular position is confirmed. A preinjection antero-posterior film is obtained at this time for subtraction purposes. Approximately 15 to 20 ml or more of contrast medium are injected in order to ensure complete filling of the joint space and suprapatellar bursa. With the needle still in place, a second anteroposterior projection is made, making sure the point of entry of the central ray is held constant. The needle is then removed and the knee exercised by passive flexion and extension. Anteroposterior, lateral, and oblique projections are made in the supine position, followed by an anteroposterior projection with traction applied to the lower leg in an effort to facilitate seepage of the contrast into areas of loosening. Subtraction radiographs are made when barium-impregnated methyl methacrylate has been used in order to better demonstrate the radioiodinated contrast medium between the bone and the methyl methacrylate.[36]

**Normal Total Knee Arthrogram.** The injected contrast medium should be confined to the joint and capsular space as well as to the suprapatellar bursa without visualization of contrast medium at the methacrylate-bone interface of the tibial component. Lym-

phatic filling may commonly be observed (Fig. 7–35).

**Abnormal Total Knee Arthrogram.** The abnormal arthrogram is indicated by contrast medium at the methacrylate-bone interface of the tibial component, indicating loosening (Fig. 7–36).

### Complications of Total Knee Arthroplasty (Table 7–2)

**Loosening.** Serial radiographs may show progressive widening of the normal lucent zone at the methacrylate-bone interface of the tibial component, confirming loosening. However, most cases necessitate arthrography for confirmation (Fig. 7–37). Radionuclide scanning may also be of value in detecting loosening of the total knee replace-

**Table 7–2.** COMPLICATIONS OF TOTAL KNEE PROSTHESES

| |
|---|
| Loosening |
| Instability or Dislocation |
| Limitation of range of motion |
| Fractures |
| Infection |

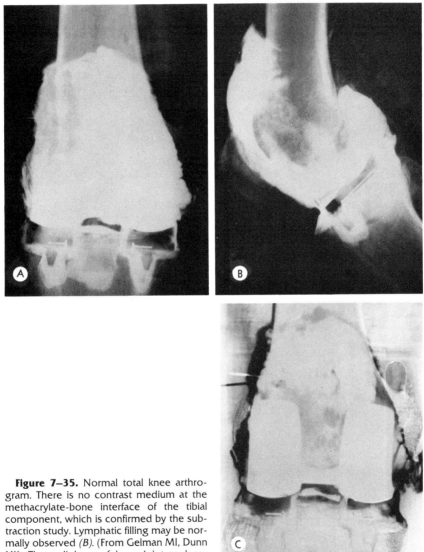

**Figure 7–35.** Normal total knee arthrogram. There is no contrast medium at the methacrylate-bone interface of the tibial component, which is confirmed by the subtraction study. Lymphatic filling may be normally observed *(B)*. (From Gelman MI, Dunn HK: The radiology of knee joint replacement. AJR *27*:447–455, 1976.)

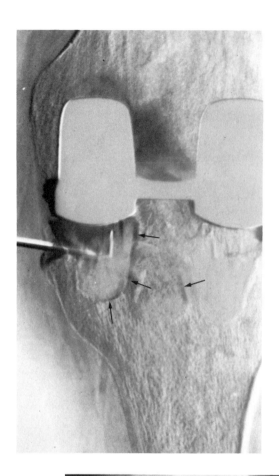

**Figure 7–36.** The abnormal total knee arthrogram. Contrast medium is present at the methacrylate-bone interface (arrows) of the tibial component, indicating loosening. (From Gelman MI, Dunn HK: The radiology of knee joint replacement. AJR 27:447–455, 1976.)

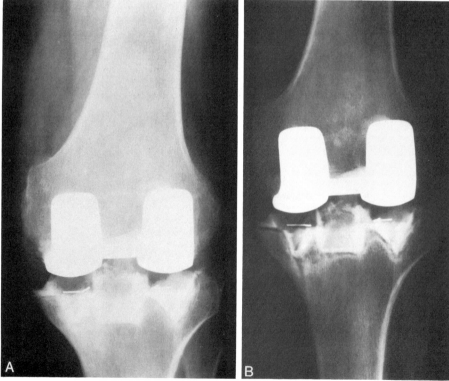

**Figure 7–37.** *A* and *B,* Interval radiographs demonstrate increased lucency at the methacrylate-bone interface of the tibial component, indicating loosening as well as fracture through the medial tibial condyle.

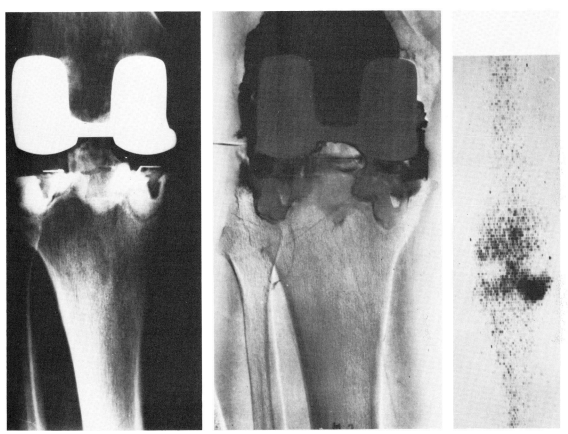

**Figure 7–38.** Radionuclide scan demonstrates increased activity in the medial tibial condyle, indicating loosening; however, the arthrogram demonstrates loosening of the tibial component in both the medial and lateral tibial condyles. (From Gelman MI, Coleman RE, Stevens PM, Davey BW: Radiography, radionuclide imaging arthrography in the evaluation of total hip and knee replacement. Radiology *128*:677–682, Sept 1978.)

ment, but at present it is probably not as dependable as for the hip (Fig. 7–38).[35]

**Instability.** Instability is usually secondary to the very lax or absent ligaments that may occur in rheumatoid arthritis and less frequently in degenerative arthritis. This instability may be corrected following total knee replacement as muscle strength increases. Persistent instability, however, may be demonstrated on weight-bearing films or fluoroscopy where stress throws the knee into varus or valgus (Fig. 7–39).

**Dislocation.** Dislocation may occur when ligamentous laxity is severe. Posterior cruciate ligamentous laxity or absence may allow hyperextension of the knee if the capsule is compromised or dislocation of the tibia with respect to the femur (Fig. 7–40).

**Limitation of Range of Motion.** Following total knee replacement, range of motion should be observable at least from 0 degrees at full extension to 90 degrees flexion. Inability to extend or flex fully with associated locking sensation may be secondary to bony impingement due to inadequate shaving of patellar or femoral osteophytes. Fluoroscopic observation and radiographic docu-

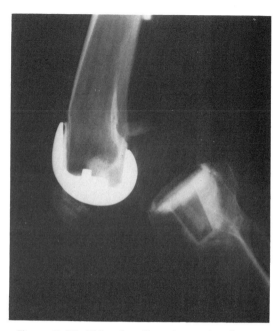

**Figure 7–40.** Dislocation. Posterior cruciate ligament and capsular laxity will allow dislocation of the tibia with a posterior drawer maneuver.

mentation will help in further evaluation (Fig. 7–41).

**Fractures.** Fracture may occur at the time of surgery or postoperatively. Manipulation during surgery may cause fracture due to marked osteoporosis. Fracture may occur postoperatively with either the hinge or resurfacing prosthesis. It is usually related to the associated osteoporosis and increased mobility, and it usually occurs in the femur (Fig. 7–42A). When hinge prostheses are used, the stress is transmitted along the metal stem and the fracture occurs in the bone immediately adjacent to the tip of the stem (Fig. 7–42B).

Malalignment of the resurfacing unit may cause fracture through the tibial plateau due to unequal distribution of stress over the tibial surface (Fig. 7–43). Supracondylar fractures may also occur, most commonly owing to the combination of osteoporotic bone and increased activity allowed by the knee prosthesis. If the prosthesis has not loosened, healing usually occurs without necessitating its removal.

Patellar fractures have been reported following total knee replacement. These are transverse in configuration and are probably due to the combined effects of osteoporosis and tension produced by quadriceps muscle contraction.[37]

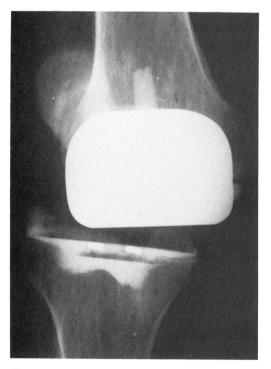

**Figure 7–39.** Instability. External rotation of the leg causes medial subluxation of the femur on the tibia owing to medial collateral ligament laxity. (From Gelman MI, Dunn HK: The radiology of knee joint replacement. AJR 27:447–455, 1976.)

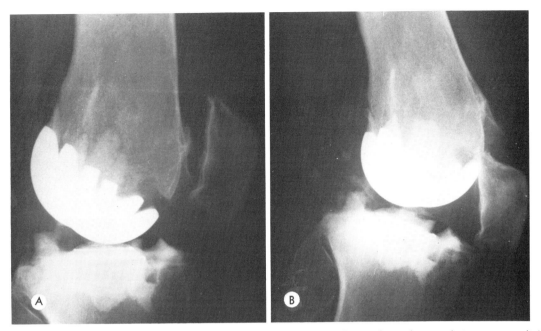

**Figure 7–41.** Limitation of range of motion. Failure to remove patellar or femoral osteophytes may result in impingement and limitation of range of motion. (From Gelman MI, Dunn HK: The radiology of knee joint replacement. AJR 27:447–455, 1976.)

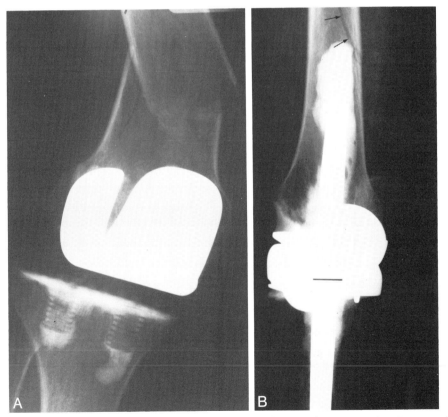

**Figure 7–42.** *A,* Supracondylar fracture may occur after total knee replacement owing to a combination of osteoporosis and increased mobility. *B,* The bone immediately adjacent to the stem of the hinge prosthesis is a common site for fracture (arrows). (Fig. 7–42*B* from Gelman MI, Dunn HK: The radiology of knee joint replacement. AJR 27:447–455, 1976.)

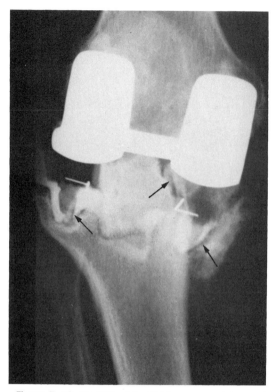

**Figure 7–43.** Fracture of the tibial component (arrows) has occurred because of malpositioning in the proximal tibia and subsequent abnormal stress concentration. (From Gelman MI, Dunn HK: The radiology of knee joint replacement. AJR 27:447–455, 1976.)

**Infection.** Infection is the major nonmechanical and most serious complication of total knee joint replacement, since it may necessitate removal of the prosthesis and possible subsequent arthrodesis (Fig. 7–44).[38] Infection may occur following postoperative hemarthrosis, and for this reason suction drains are used in the immediate postoperative period. Chronic infection, which may exist in the rheumatoid joint and go undetected prior to joint replacement surgery, can be confused with infection caused by the prosthesis. The radiographic manifestations of infection include soft tissue swelling and loosening, and less commonly, bony destruction (Fig. 7–45). Arthrography is useful in demonstrating loosening, and a sample of the joint fluid should be sent to the laboratory for aerobic and anaerobic culture to ensure the absence of infection whenever arthrography is done.

Arthrodesis, or knee fusion, has been used to stabilize the knee and correct deformity following polio, as well as the sequelae of

pigmented villonodular synovitis, hemophilia, tuberculosis, and pyogenic septic arthritis (Fig. 7–46). It is also utilized in selective cases of rheumatoid, degenerative, and posttraumatic arthritis not meeting the criteria for total knee replacement.[39] Bony ankylosis may also occur spontaneously following severe rheumatoid arthritis (Fig. 7–47).

**Acquired or Developmental Deformity.** Angular deformities of the knee such as genu varum (bowlegs) or genu valgum (knock-knees) may be corrected prior to closure of the growth plates by stapling one side of the growth plate and allowing the opposite side to continue to grow and effect the correction. The medial aspect of the growth plate is stapled to correct a knock-knee deformity, while stapling of the lateral aspect is utilized to correct a bowleg deformity. The body of the staple should be perpendicular to the growth plate and in contact with the surface of the bone. The legs of the staple should point toward the axis of the bone and be equidistant from the epiphyseal plate (Fig. 7–48). If the growth plate has already closed,

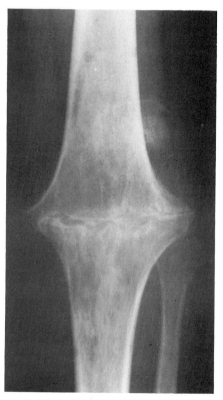

**Figure 7–44.** Arthrodesis was performed following infected total knee prosthesis in patients with rheumatoid arthritis.

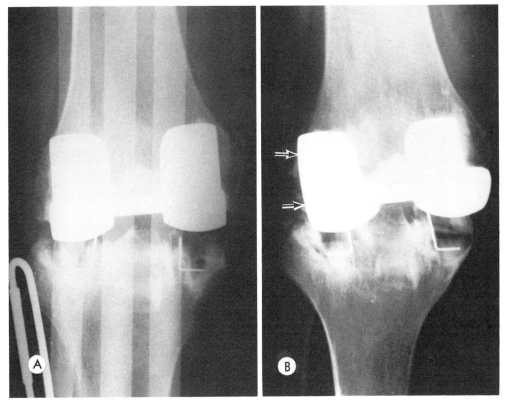

**Figure 7–45.** Infected total knee prosthesis with bony destruction (arrows) over interval between *(A)* and *(B)*. (From Gelman MI, Dunn HK: The radiology of knee joint replacement. AJR *27*:447–455, 1976.)

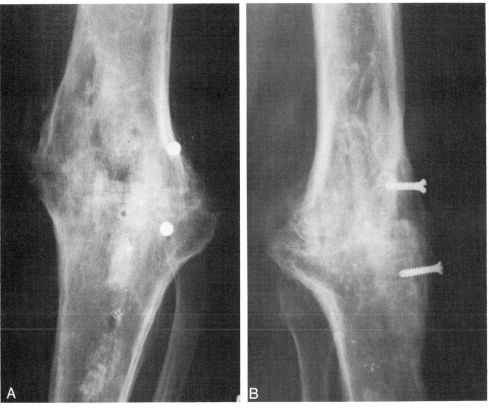

**Figure 7–46.** *A* and *B*, Knee arthrodesis following septic arthritis of the knee.

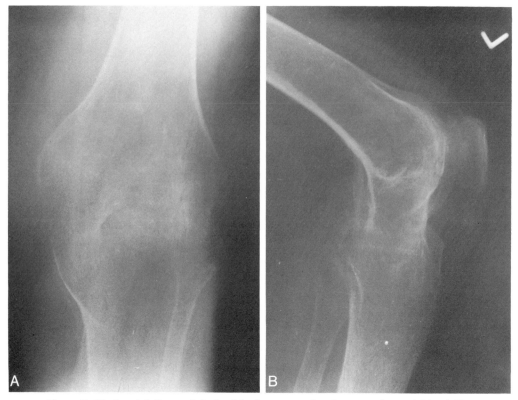

**Figure 7–47.** *A* and *B*, Bony ankylosis of the knee secondary to severe rheumatoid arthritis.

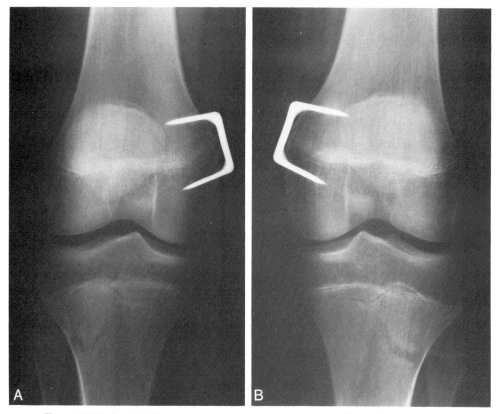

**Figure 7–48.** *A* and *B*, Staple procedure to correct genu valgum (knock knee deformity).

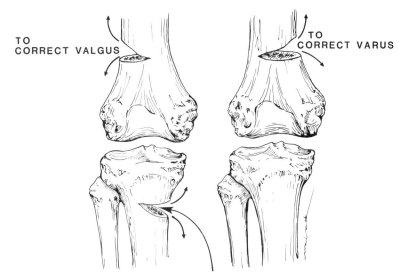

**Figure 7–49.** Opening wedge osteotomy for correction of genu varum and genu valgum deformity.

correction of developmental or post-trau-matic angular deformity may be accom-plished by an opening wedge osteotomy at the site of greatest deformity, either in the distal femur or the proximal tibia (Fig. 7–49). Genu recurvatum deformity, or hyper-extension of the knee joint (due to trauma resulting in decreased development of the anterior aspect of the distal femoral or prox-imal tibial epiphyseal growth plate), may be corrected surgically by an opening wedge osteotomy of the anterior aspect of the prox-imal tibia (Fig. 7–50).[34]

Patellar dislocation or subluxation may be facilitated by a genu valgum deformity of the knee, an underdeveloped lateral femoral condyle or patellar groove on the femur, or an elongated patellar tendon as evidenced by a high-riding patella (patella alta) on the lateral view (Fig. 7–51). Radiographic as-

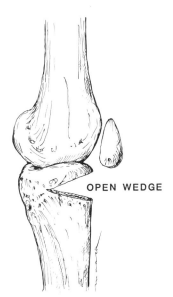

**Figure 7–50.** Opening wedge osteotomy for correc-tion of genu recurvatum deformity.

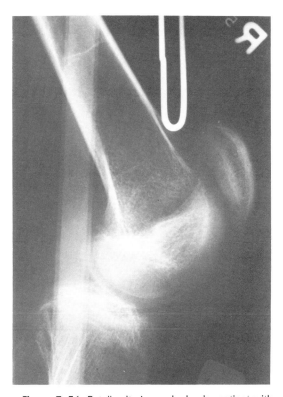

**Figure 7–51.** Patella alta in cerebral palsy patient with flexion contracture.

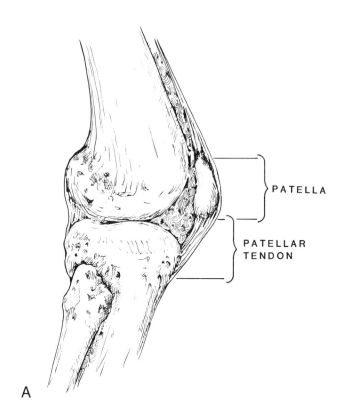

PATELLA

PATELLAR
TENDON

A

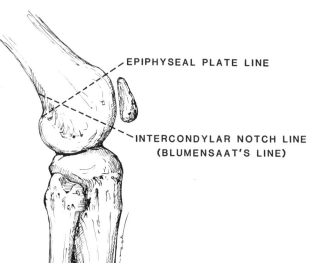

EPIPHYSEAL PLATE LINE

INTERCONDYLAR NOTCH LINE
(BLUMENSAAT'S LINE)

B

**Figure 7–52.** Proper positioning of patella may be assessed by patella-patellar tendon ratio *(A)*. Ratio of length of patella to patellar tendon length should equal 1–1.1. *B,* Patella should lie between the epiphyseal plate line and the intercondylar notch line (Blumensaat's line) with the knee in 30 degrees of flexion.

sessment of high-riding patella may be made by determining the patella–patellar tendon ratio or the relationship of the patella to the former epiphyseal plate line and Bloomensaat's line (Fig. 7–52).[40] Subluxation of the patella is indicated on the tangential view by lateral tilting, resulting in displacement of the lateral edge of the patella lateral to the lateral femoral condyle while the apex of the patella is displaced out of the intercondylar notch of the femur (Fig. 7–53).[41] Occasionally, complete dislocation may occur that is appreciated only on the tangential view (Fig. 7–54). Because of the variability associated with degree of flexion of the knee and position of the patella on tangential view, the technique proposed by Merchant[42] provides greater objectivity in measurement of lateral subluxation of the patella and hy-

poplasia of the femoral condyle. Surgical correction of recurrent dislocation or subluxation may be effected by transplantation of the tibial tubercle and attached patellar tendon medially and distally (Hauser procedure) (see Figs. 7–33 and 7–55). Overcorrection may result in excessive pain and limitation of motion due to a low-lying patella (patella baja).[45]

Chondromalacia, or softening of the articular cartilage of the patella, may be idiopathic or may result from repeated episodes of trauma, subluxation or dislocation, increased valgus deformity of the knee, or patella alta (high-lying patella). Plain films usually show the bone to be normal, but patellar malalignment consisting of lateral subluxation and patella alta can be seen, as can sclerosis of the posterior aspect of the

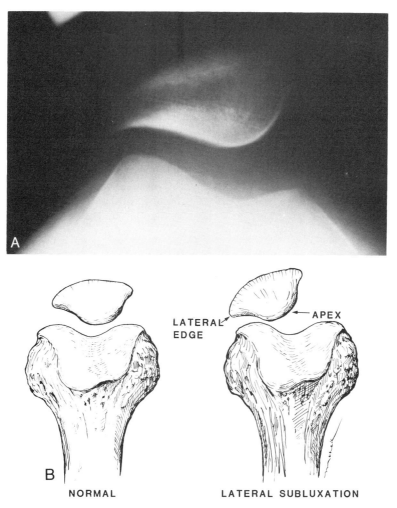

**Figure 7–53.** Lateral subluxation of the patella is radiographically characterized by lateral tilting of the patella and displacement of the apex of the patella out of the intercondylar notch of the femur.

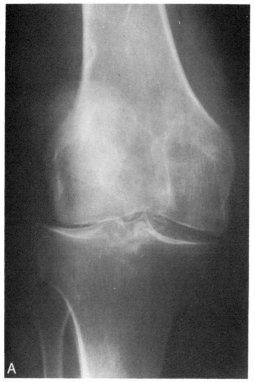
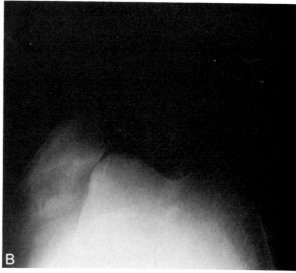

**Figure 7–54.** *A* and *B*, Lateral dislocation of the patella is best illustrated on the tangential view.

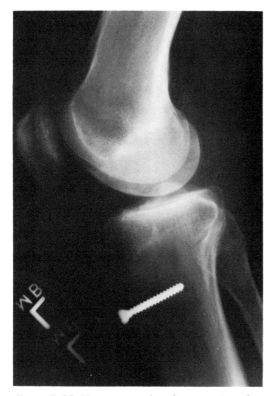

**Figure 7–55.** Houser procedure for correction of recurrent dislocation or subluxation of the patella.

patella, patellofemoral joint space narrowing, and fracture or degenerative spurring on the lateral margin of the patella.[46] Infrequently, arthrography may demonstrate chondromalacia. Treatment may include shaving the patellar cartilage, patellar tendon transplantation, or patellectomy.

## References

1. Hohl M, Larson RL: Fractures and dislocation of the knee. *In* Rockwood CA, Green DP (eds): Fractures. Vol 2. J. B. Lippincott Co., Philadelphia, 1975, pp. 1131–1284
2. Hohl M: Tibial condylar fractures. J Bone Joint Surg 49A:1455–1467, 1967
3. Newberg AH, Greenstein R: Radiographic evaluation of tibial plateau fractures. Radiology 126:319–323, 1978
4. Elstrom J, Pankovich AM, Sasson H, Rodriguez J: The use of tomography in the assessment of fractures of the tibial plateau. J Bone Joint Surg 58A:551–555, 1976
5. Apley AG: Fractures of the tibial plateau. Orthop Clin N Am 10:61–74, 1979
6. Pavlov H, Freiberger RH, Deck MF, Marshall JL, Morrissey JK: Computer-assisted tomography of the knee. Invest Radiol 13:57–62, 1978
7. Archer CR, Yeager V: Internal structures of the knee visualized by computed tomography. J Comput Assist Tomogr 2:181–183, 1978

8. DaLinka MK, Gohel VK, Rancier L: Tomography in the evaluation of the anterior cruciate ligament. Radiology 108:31–33, 1973
9. Giles D, Gelman MI, Rosenberg TD: The anterior tibial plateau mound sign: an arthrographic sign of complete anterior cruciate ligament disruption. Personal communication.
10. Nicoll EA: Fractures of the tibial shaft. A survey of 705 cases. J Bone Joint Surg 46B:373–387, 1964
11. Nelson G, Kelly P, Peterson L, Jones T: Blood supply of the human tibia. J Bone Joint Surg 42A:625–635, 1960
12. Urist MR, Mazet R Jr, McLean FC: The pathogenesis and treatment of delayed union and nonunion, a survey of eighty-five ununited fractures of the shaft of the tibia and one hundred control cases with similar injuries. J Bone Joint Surg 36A:931–967, 1954
13. Broun PW, Urban JG: Early weight-bearing treatment of open fractures of the tibia. J Bone Joint Surg 51A:59–75, 1969
14. Pierce RO: Complications of traction, plaster and appliances. In Epps CH (ed): Complications in Orthopaedic Surgery. Vol. 1. J. B. Lippincott Co., Philadelphia, 1978, p. 82
15. Fernandez-Palazzi F: Fibular resection in delayed union of tibial fractures. Acta Orthop Scand 40:105–118, 1969
16. Kenmore PI, Kramik AD: Complication of musculoskeletal infection. In Epps CH, (ed.): Complications in Orthopaedic Surgery. Vol. 1. J. B. Lippincott Co., Philadelphia, 1978, pp. 129–158
17. Kunkel WG, Lynn RB: The anterior tibial compartment syndrome. Canad J Surg 1:212–217, 1958
18. Sorenson KH: Treatment of delayed union and nonunion of the tibia by fibular resection. Acta Orthop Scand 40:92–104, 1969
19. Huntington TW: Case of bone transference. Use of a segment of fibula to supply a defect in the tibia. Ann Surg 41:249–251, 1905
20. Codinilla A: On the care of congenital pseudoarthrosis of the tibia by means of periosteal transplantation. Am J Orthop Surg 4:163–169, 1906
21. McMaster PE, Hahl M: Tibiofibular cross-peg grafting. J Bone Joint Surg 47A:1146–1158, 1965
22. Campanacci M, Zanoli S: Double tibiofibular synostosis for nonunion and delayed union of the tibia. J Bone Joint Surg 48A:44–56, 1966
23. Shelton ML, Anderson RL: Complications of fractures and dislocations of the ankle. In Epps CH (ed.): Complications in Orthopaedic Surgery. Vol. I. J. B. Lippincott Co., Philadelphia, 1978, pp. 535–577
24. Fairbank TJ: Knee joint changes after meniscectomy. J Bone Joint Surg 30B:664–670, 1948
25. Huckell J: Is meniscectomy a benign procedure? A long-term follow-up study. Canad J Surg 8:254–260, 1965
26. Tapper EM, Hover NW: Late results after meniscectomy. J Bone Joint Surg 51A:517–526, 1969
27. Dandy DJ: The diagnosis of problems after meniscectomy. J Bone Joint Surg 57B:349–352, 1975
28. Milgram JW: Radiological and pathological manifestations of osteochondritis dissecans of the distal femur. A study of 50 cases. Radiology 126:305–311, 1978
29. Milgram JW, Rogers LF, Miller JW: Osteochondral fractures: mechanisms of injury and fate of fragments. AJR 130:651–658, 1978
30. Gilley JS, Gelman MI, Edson DM, Metcalf RW: Chondral fractures of the knee: arthrographic, arthroscopic and clinical manifestations. Radiology 138:51–54, 1981
31. Coventry MB: Osteotomy of the upper portion of the tibia for degenerative arthritis of the knee. J Bone Joint Surg 47A:984–990, 1965
32. Conventry MB: Osteotomy about the knee for degenerative and rheumatoid arthritis. J Bone Joint Surg 55A:23–48, 1973
33. Coventry MB: Upper tibial osteotomy for gonarthrosis. Orthop Clin N Am 10:191–210, 1979
34. Turek SL: Orthopaedics: Principles and their Application. 3rd ed. J. B. Lippincott Co., 1977, pp. 1137–1244
35. Gelman, MI, Coleman RE, Stevens PM, Davey BW: Radiography, radionuclide imaging, and arthrography in the evaluation of total hip and knee replacement. Radiology 128:677–682, 1978
36. Gelman MI, Dunn HK: Radiology of knee joint replacement. AJR 127:447–455, 1976
37. Freeman MAR, Hammer A: Patellar fracture after replacement of the tibia-femoral joint with the ICLH prosthesis. Arch Orthop Trauma Surg 92:63–67, 1978
38. Laskin RS: Total knee replacement. Orthop Clin N Am 10:223–247, 1979
39. Dee R: The case for arthrodesis of the knee. Orthop Clin N Am 10:249–261, 1979
40. Insall J, Salvati E: Patella position in the normal knee joint. Radiology 101:101–104, 1971
41. Hughston JA: Subluxation of the patella. J Bone Joint Surg. 50A: 1003–1026, 1968
42. Merchant AC, Mercer RL, Jacobsen RH, Cool CR: Roentgenographic analysis of patella-femoral congruence. J Bone Joint Surg 56A:1391–1396, 1974
43. Chrisman OD, Snook GA, Wilson TC: A long term prospective study of the Hauser and Roux-Goldthwait procedure for recurrent patellar dislocation. Clin Orthop Rel Res 144:27–30, 1979
44. Fiedling JW, Liebler WA, Krishne Urs ND, Wilson SA, Puglisi AS: Tibial tubercle transfer. A long-range follow-up study. Clin Orthop Rel Res 144:43–44, 1979
45. Blazina ME, Fox JM, Carlson GJ, Jurgutis JJ: Patella baja. J Bone Joint Surg 57A:1027, 1975
46. Gruber MA: The conservative treatment of chondromalacia patellae. Orthop Clin N Am 10:105–115, 1979

# 8

---

# THE ANKLE AND FOOT

The ankle and foot are most often evaluated radiologically and orthopedically for traumatic, congenital, and acquired conditions. This area may be somewhat confusing to the radiologist because of the orthopedic terms used to describe the various conditions as well as unfamiliarity that comes because these entities are not seen often. In contrast, the orthopedic surgeon has a good idea of what he is dealing with based on clinical history and physical examination and orders the radiographs to confirm a diagnosis as well as for use as a baseline for any subsequent orthopedic procedure, and thus to assess improvement of anatomic alignment.

## TRAUMATIC CONDITIONS

Significant bony trauma to the ankle may be demonstrated by anteroposterior, lateral, and 20-degree internal oblique projections for the mortise. Widening of the tibial-fibular syndesmosis greater than 3 mm indicates diastasis, whereas shift of the talus in the absence of bony fracture on the widened side indicates ligamentous rupture. Stress views help in identifying complete or incomplete ligamentous tears (sprains) as well as demonstrating ligamentous injury when the plain films are normal (Figs. 8–1 and 8–2). The lateral collateral ligament, more frequently torn than the medial (deltoid) ligament, includes the anterior talofibular ligament, the posterior talofibular ligament, and the calcaneofibular ligament (Fig. 8–3). Of these, the anterior talofibular ligament is most commonly torn, followed by the cal-

caneofibular ligament. Because only one of these ligaments may be more affected than the others, anteroposterior varus (inversion) stress views with the foot in plantar flexion are recommended so that isolated ligamentous tears can be more effectively recognized. Widening of the tibiotalar joint laterally seen with the foot in plantar flexion but not seen with the foot in a neutral position indicates anterior talofibular ligament disruption. Lateral tibiotalar widening in both the plantar flexion and neutral positions, on the other hand, indicates anterior talofibular and calcaneofibular ligament disruption.[1]

Anterior subluxation of the talus on the lateral view with the foot in plantar flexion indicates anterior talofibular ligament injury[2] (Fig. 8–4) (Table 8–1).

Comparison views of the opposite side should be included because of the wide range of normal variation between patients. Apparently, there may even be variation between ankles in the same patient.[3]

Arthrography may be useful in demonstrating anterior talofibular, calcaneofibular, and deltoid ligament tears, but it must be done shortly after the injury to prevent false negatives resulting from fibrin or clot occluding the tear and preventing extravasation of the contrast medium[4] (Fig. 8–5).

The necessity and usefulness of the arthrogram is determined mainly by the philosophy of the orthopedic surgeon regarding surgical repair of acute ligamentous injuries. Usually, stretched ligaments are treated by immobilization, while complete disruption may or may not be treated by surgical repair. Assessment of whether or not the ligament

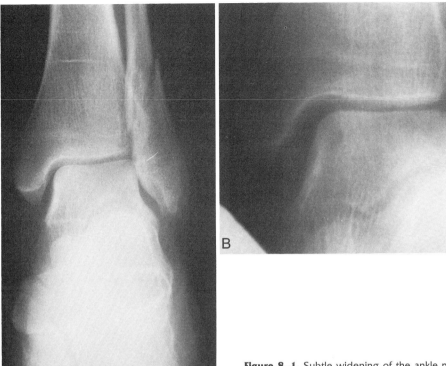

**Figure 8–1.** Subtle widening of the ankle mortice medially on a plain film *(A)* is confirmed by stress view *(B),* made under fluoroscopy, indicating a deltoid ligament tear.

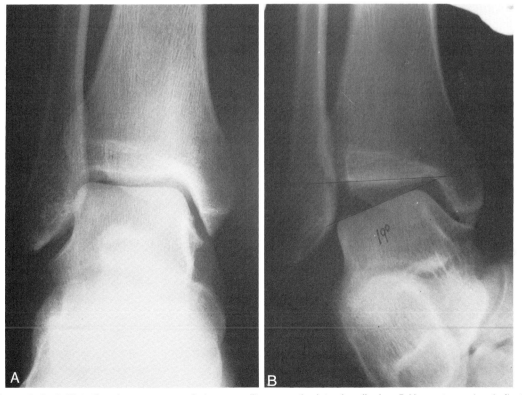

**Figure 8–2.** *A,* Plain film demonstrates soft tissue swelling over the lateral malleolus. *B,* Varus stress view indicates lateral ligament instability.

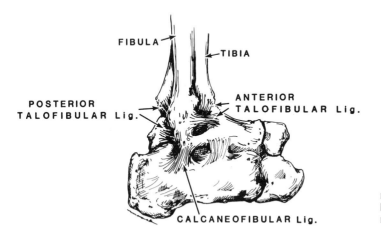

FIBULA

TIBIA

POSTERIOR
TALOFIBULAR Lig.

ANTERIOR
TALOFIBULAR Lig.

CALCANEOFIBULAR Lig.

**Figure 8–3.** The lateral collateral ligament consists of the anterior talofibular
ligament, the posterior talofibular ligament, and the calcaneofibular ligament.

**Table 8–1.** STRESS VIEWS DEMONSTRATING THE MORE COMMON LIGAMENTOUS
INJURIES OF THE ANKLE

| View | Observation | Injury |
|---|---|---|
| Anteroposterior varus stress view | Widened tibiotalar joint laterally with foot in plantar flexion | Anterior talofibular ligament disruption |
| | or | |
| | No widening of tibiotalar joint laterally with foot in neutral position | |
| Lateral view | Anterior subluxation of talus with foot in plantar flexion | Anterior talofibular ligament disruption |
| Anteroposterior varus stress view | Widened tibiotalar joint laterally with foot in plantar flexion | Anterior talofibular ligament disruption |
| | or | |
| | Widening of tibiotalar joint laterally with foot in neutral position | Calcaneofibular ligament disruption |

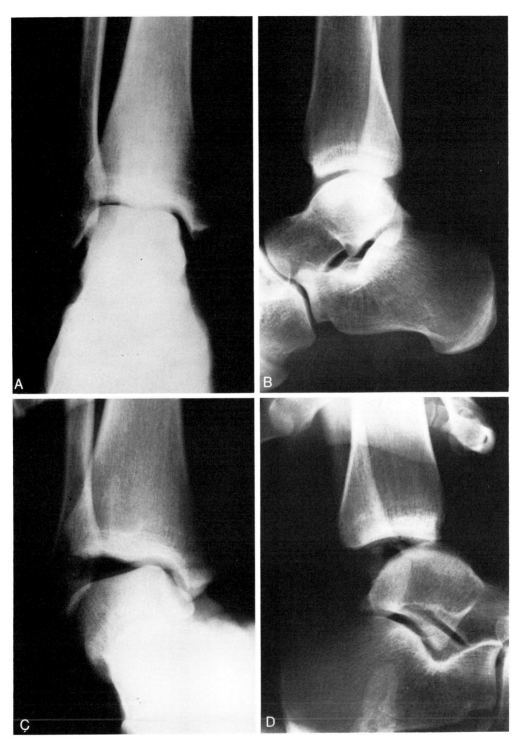

**Figure 8–4.** *A* and *B*, Nonstress views give no indication that ligamentous injury has occurred. *C* and *D*, Widening of the tibiotalar joint laterally in both neutral and plantar flexion positions indicates anterior talofibular and calcaneofibular ligament injury, whereas anterior subluxation of the talus indicates anterior talofibular ligament injury.

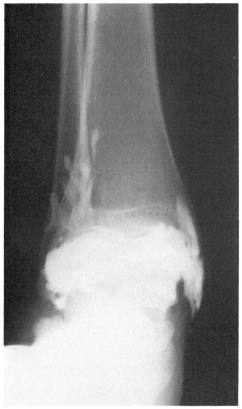

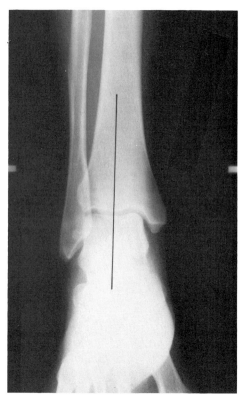

**Figure 8–6.** Assessment of anatomic position of the tibiotalar joint. A line drawn through the midaxis of the tibia should pass through the midaxis of the talus.

**Figure 8–5.** Arthrogram demonstrates tears in the deltoid ligament and the tibiofibular syndesmosis.

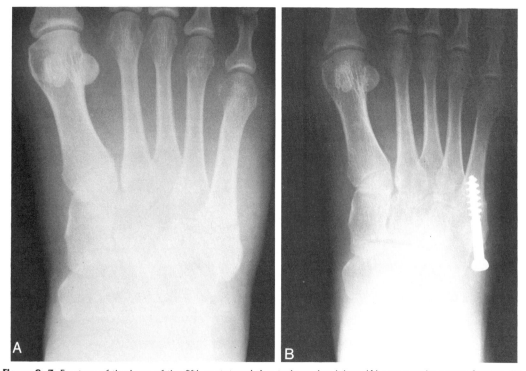

**Figure 8–7.** Fracture of the base of the fifth metatarsal due to inversion injury *(A)* may require screw fixation *(B)*.

is completely disrupted, therefore, may be delayed after a trial of immobilization, rendering the arthrogram a less useful and effective diagnostic modality.[5]

In evaluating postreduction films of trauma to the ankle, the criteria utilized for adequate reduction include anatomic position of the talus beneath the tibial plafond (Fig. 8–6), a smooth articular surface, and a joint line parallel to the ground. In approximately 10 per cent of cases of talar dislocation, reduction is prevented by ligamentous or posterior tibial tendon displacement into the joint, necessitating operative intervention.[6]

Metatarsal fractures are usually treated by closed reduction with a cast. Fractures of the base of the fifth metatarsal (Jones fracture) due to an inversion injury with pulling on the peroneus brevis tendon may require internal fixation for stabilization (Fig. 8–7). These fractures may frequently be detected on a lateral view of the ankle when an ankle injury is suspected clinically.

Calcaneal fractures vary in extent as well as in method of treatment (treatment without

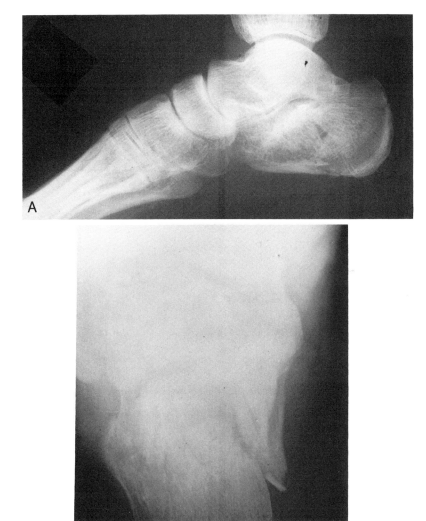

**Figure 8–8.** Lateral (A) and tangential (B) views of the calcaneus demonstrate extension of fracture through the sustentaculum tali. Since a portion of the deltoid ligament attaches here, this type of injury renders the ankle more unstable.

reduction, closed reduction, open reduction, or primary subtalar or triple arthrodesis), depending on the approach of the orthopedic surgeon. Lateral and tangential views best demonstrate calcaneal fractures, and, if the fracture extends through the sustentaculum tali medially, this renders the ankle more unstable, since the deltoid ligament partially inserts on this structure (Fig. 8–8). Complications of these fractures include subtalar post-traumatic arthritis requiring a triple arthrodesis and stenosing tenosynovitis of the peroneal tendons due to impingement.[7, 8]

This impingement may be demonstrated by peroneal tenography whereby 10 to 20 ml of Renografin 60 are injected under fluoroscopic control into the common peroneal tendon sheath above the lateral malleolus using a 1.5 inch 22 gauge needle. Anteroposterior, lateral, and oblique views as well as an anteroposterior view with the forefoot in inversion and the beam angled 45 degrees cephalad are obtained. The abnormal peroneal tenogram demonstrates lateral displacement or compression of the peroneal tendon[9, 10] (Fig. 8–9).

Fractures of the talus vary in severity and may be complicated by avascular necrosis. Treatment for these more severe fractures include tibial calcaneal fusion after removal of the talus or a pantalar arthrodesis (tibiotalar, talocalcaneal, talonavicular, and calcaneocuboid fusion). Radiographic evidence of fusion is usually observed by 16 to 20 weeks postoperatively; however, pseudarthrosis may result. Acute osteochondral fractures of the talus are most commonly observed on the lateral aspect of the articular surface of the talus and must be distinguished from osteochondritis dissecans, which occurs on the medial aspect of the articular surface. These fractures may heal or detach and become loose body fragments or they may not heal, in which case surgical removal is usually required (Fig. 8–10).[11–15]

Unstable injuries such as bimalleolar or trimalleolar fractures or a malleolar fracture with avulsion of the contralateral ligament usually require open reduction and internal fixation (Fig. 8–11).

Nonunion of a medial malleolus fracture is more common than in a lateral or posterior malleolus fracture and necessitates screw fixation. Disruption of the syndesmosis also requires internal fixation for stabilization (Fig. 8–12).

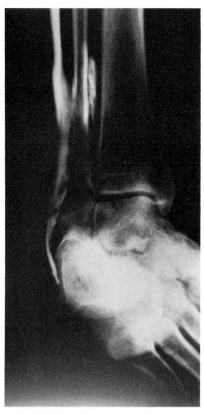

**Figure 8–9.** Peroneal tenogram demonstrating stenosing peroneal tenosynovitis following a calcaneal fracture. Note the abrupt cutoff of contrast medium in the distal aspect of the peroneal tendon.

Post-traumatic arthritis, which occurs in 20 to 40 per cent of ankle fractures, is radiographically manifested by joint space narrowing, subchondral sclerosis, eburnation, and hypertrophic spurring, and it may necessitate arthrodesis or total joint arthroplasty (Fig. 8–13).[16–18]

## ARTHRITIS

Rheumatoid arthritis or post-traumatic degenerative arthritis of the tibiotalar or subtalar joints may be treated by arthrodesis or, in selected cases, by a resurfacing prosthesis (Fig. 8–14). These are subject to the same complications that occur with total joint prostheses in other joints, including instability, loosening, fracture, and infection.[19]

Metatarsophalangeal subluxation commonly occurs in rheumatoid arthritis, resulting in pronation of the metatarsal heads with subsequent disruption of the skin over these pressure points. Metatarsal head oste-

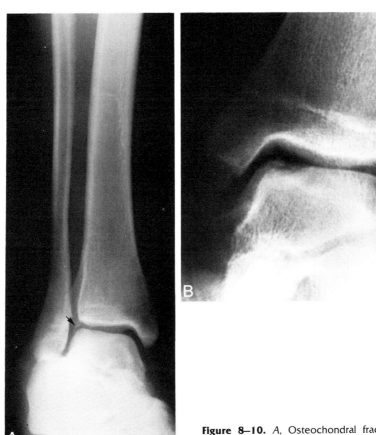

**Figure 8–10.** *A*, Osteochondral fracture of the talus (arrow). *B*, Osteochondritis dissecans.

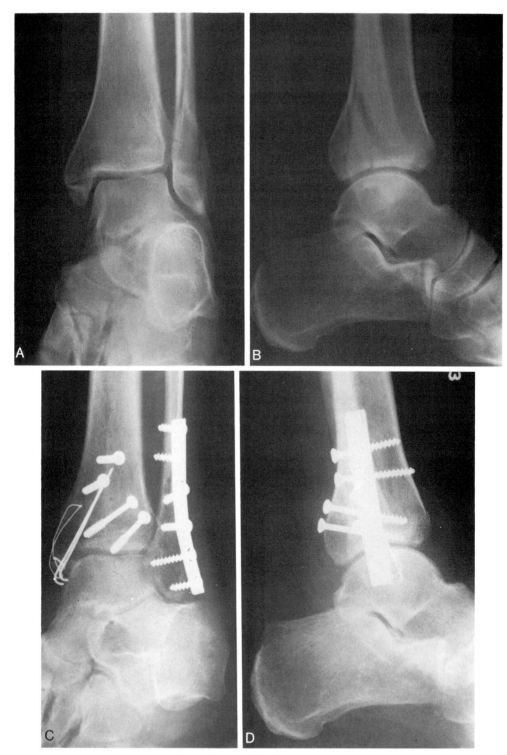

**Figure 8–11.** Trimalleolar fracture (*A* and *B*) with subsequent internal fixation (*C* and *D*).

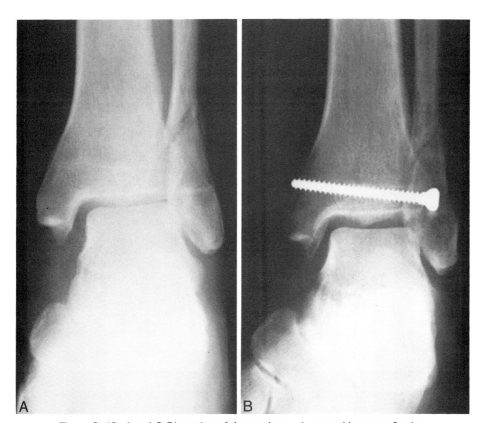

**Figure 8–12.** *A* and *B*, Disruption of the syndesmosis treated by screw fixation.

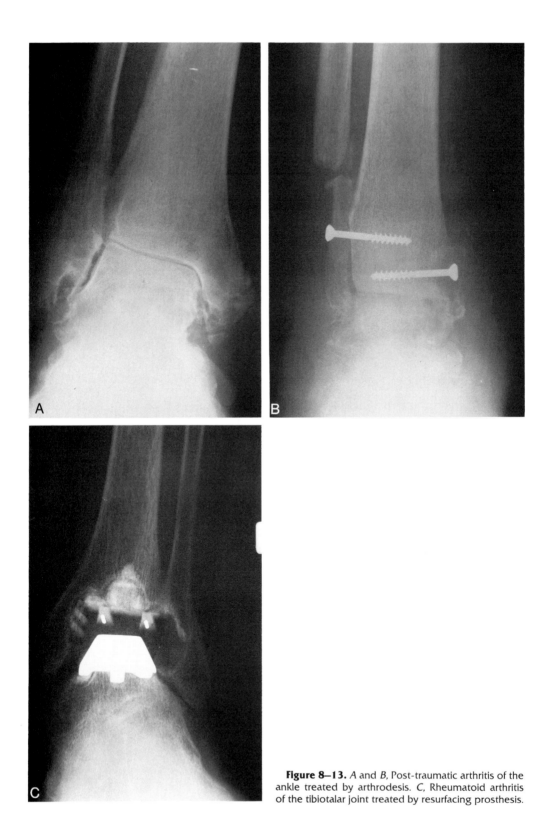

**Figure 8–13.** *A* and *B*, Post-traumatic arthritis of the ankle treated by arthrodesis. *C*, Rheumatoid arthritis of the tibiotalar joint treated by resurfacing prosthesis.

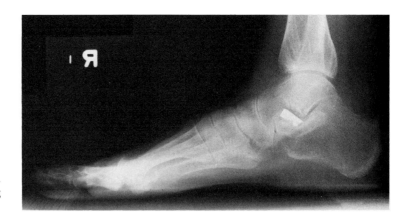

**Figure 8–14.** Post-traumatic subtalar arthritis treated by resurfacing prosthesis.

otomy (Stone-Hoffman procedure) may be performed to eliminate the pressure points. In addition, hyperextension and flexion deformities of the toes may be corrected by pin fixation (Fig. 8–15).

## CONGENITAL DEFORMITIES

An understanding of congenital deformities of the foot requires an understanding and familiarity with the following specific terms and definitions:[20]

*Hindfoot*: talus and calcaneus.

*Forefoot*: tarsal bones, metatarsals, and phalanges.

*Clubfoot*: Congenital or acquired malformation of the foot, most commonly talipes equinovarus.

*Talipes*: congenital deformity of the foot.

*Pes*: acquired condition, e.g., pes planus, pes cavus.

*Varus*: medial deviation.

*Valgus*: lateral deviation.

*Equinus*: plantar flexion of the foot.

*Calcaneus*: dorsiflexion of the foot.

*Cavus*: elevation of the longitudinal arch.

*Planus*: flattening of the longitudinal arch.

Since weight-bearing views are mandatory in order to assess axial alignment of the feet, corresponding views may be obtained in the infant by maintaining firm pressure of the foot against the film in the anteroposterior projection and against a block of wood in the lateral projection, allowing future reproducibility.

Knowledge of the normal axial relationships of the bones of the foot is required in order to recognize abnormal states. This does not mean measurements must be made in every instance, but rather in those situations where the deformity is subtle or postoperative correction is being assessed. In order to keep measurements to a minimum, the following film views are recommended:

**Anteroposterior Weight-Bearing Projection.** A line drawn through the longitudinal axis of the talus should extend through the longitudinal axis of the first metatarsal.

A line drawn through the longitudinal axis of the calcaneus should extend through the longitudinal axis of the fourth metatarsal or between the fourth and fifth metatarsals.

The angle of the apex formed by the intersection of these two lines (talocalcaneal angle) should be 15 to 35 degrees (Table 8–2) (Fig. 8–16).

**Lateral Weight-Bearing Projection.** A line drawn through the longitudinal axis of the talus extends through the longitudinal axis of the first metatarsal.

A line drawn through the longitudinal axis of the calcaneus or tangential to its inferior margin intersects the talar–first metatarsal

**Table 8–2.** RELATIONSHIP OF ANGLES IN ANTEROPOSTERIOR VIEW TO DEFORMITY OF FOOT

| | | Forefoot | Hindfoot |
|---|---|---|---|
| ↑ Talocalcaneal angle | | | Valgus |
| ↓ Talocalcaneal angle | | | Varus |
| Medial alignment ⎤ | | Varus or adduction | |
| ⎬ 1st & 4th metatarsals | | | |
| Lateral alignment ⎦ | | Valgus or abduction | |

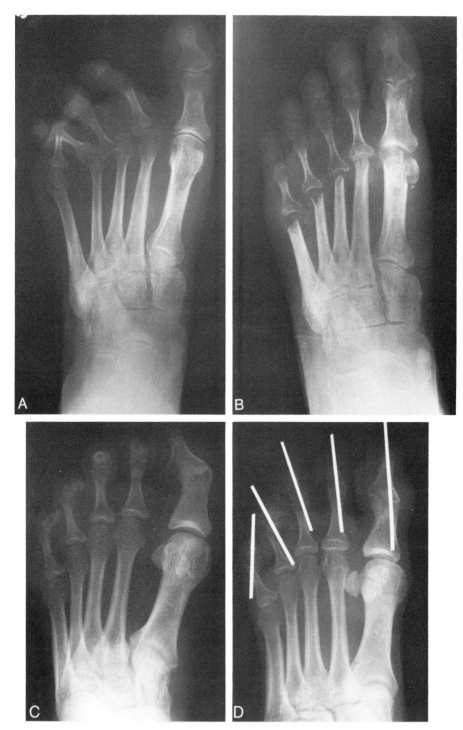

**Figure 8–15.** Stone-Hoffman procedure. Pronation deformities of metatarsal phalangeal joints *(A)* are treated by subsequent metatarsal head resections *(B)*. *C* and *D,* Correction of flexion deformities of the toes by pin fixation.

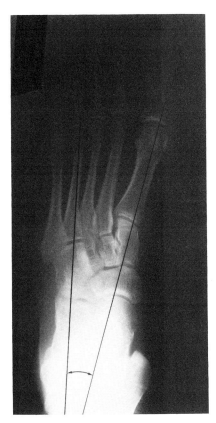

**Figure 8–16.** Measurements made on the anteroposterior weight-bearing view of the foot include midtalar line, midcalcaneal line, and talocalcaneal angle.

line making a talocalcaneal angle of 15 to 35 degrees (Table 8–3) (Fig. 8–17).[21]

## Congenital Clubfoot (Talipes Equinovarus)

In the anteroposterior projection there is a decreased talocalcaneal angle (hindfoot varus) and forefoot varus (Fig. 8–18). The lateral projection shows a decreased talocalcaneal angle (hindfoot varus).

**Table 8–3.** RELATIONSHIP OF ANGLES IN LATERAL VIEW TO DEFORMITY OF FOOT

|  | Hindfoot |
| --- | --- |
| ↑ Talocalcaneal angle | Valgus |
| ↓ Talocalcaneal angle | Varus |

Surgical treatment, implemented when more conservative manipulation and casting is not successful, consists predominantly of soft tissue releases about the foot and ankle (posterior, medial, and subtalar). Postoperative radiographic evaluation of the result necessitates a lateral view with the foot held in maximum dorsiflexion. Inadequate dorsiflexion of the anterior aspect of the talus, persistent parallelism of the talus and calcaneus, and absence of the normal overlap of the anterior aspect of the calcaneus and talus indicate incomplete correction despite the apparent normal appearance on the anteroposterior view.

Complications of therapy include "rockerbottom" flat foot and "flat-topped" talus due to avascular necrosis.[22]

Clubfoot deformity that results in fixed bony changes requires bone resection and triple arthrodesis.

## Congenital Metatarsus Adductus (Metatarsus Varus)

In the anteroposterior projection adduction or sharp medial angulation of the metatarsals is seen at the tarsometatarsal joints (Fig. 8–19). Treatment consists of manipulation and casts.

## Congenital Vertical Talus

In the lateral projection the talus is vertical and almost perpendicular to the weight-

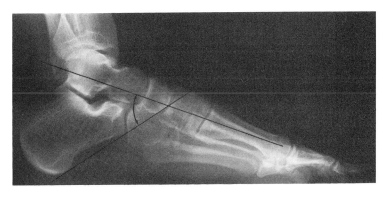

**Figure 8–17.** Measurements made on the lateral weight-bearing view of the foot include midtalar line, midcalcaneal line, and talocalcaneal angle.

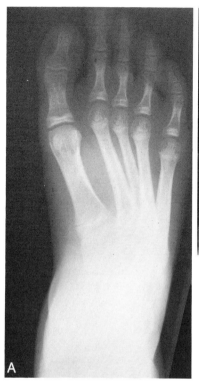

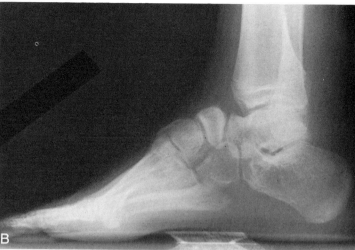

**Figure 8–18.** Congenital club foot (talipes equinovarus).

bearing surface (Fig. 8–20). In the anteroposterior projection there is an increased talocalcaneal angle (hindfoot valgus, forefoot valgus). Treatment consists of soft tissue releases and maintenance of talonavicular reduction by casting.[23, 24]

## Congenital Hallux Varus

This deformity is characterized by medial angulation of the great toe at the metatarsophalangeal joint (Fig. 8–21). Treatment consists of removal of bone from the lateral aspect of the head of the first metatarsal, removal of the accessory bone and the medial sesamoid, freeing up of the capsule, and rerouting the tendon of the extensor hallucis brevis muscle.

## ACQUIRED CONDITIONS

### Hallux Valgus

Hallux valgus is a deformity of the great toe that may have multiple different causes, such as heredity, narrow shoes, degenerative arthritis of the first metatarsophalangeal joint, and flatfoot.

The deformity consists of medial angula-

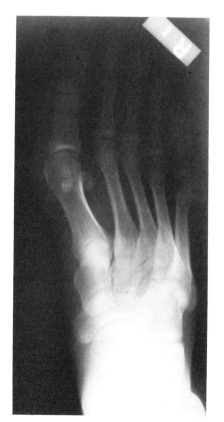

**Figure 8–19.** Congenital metatarsus varus (metatarsus adductus) is characterized by medial angulation of the metatarsals.

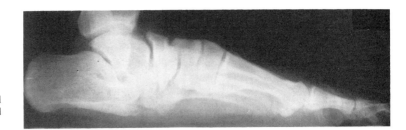

**Figure 8–20.** Congenital vertical talus is characterized by the vertical orientation of the talus.

tion of the first metatarsal, lateral angulation of the proximal phalanx, and lateral displacement of the sesamoids (Fig. 8–22). Degenerative changes that may or may not be observed at the first metatarsophalangeal joint, result in a narrowed and rigid joint (hallux rigidus).

Treatment is surgical and consists of soft tissue or bone excision procedures. Soft tissue correction employs freeing up of tendons and reimplanting them in order to correct muscle imbalance and alignment (McBride procedure). Bone excision procedures are necessary when the deformity has progressed to fixed bony changes.

Hemiarthroplasty of the first metatarsophalangeal joint involves resection of the proximal half of the proximal phalanx (Keller procedure) and partial resection of the metatarsal head (Fig. 8–23).[25–28]

Osteotomy of the proximal, middle, or distal portion of the metatarsal corrects the varus deformity (metatarsus primus varus) (Fig. 8–24).[29, 30]

Osteotomy of the proximal phalanx is performed to relieve the valgus deformity of the great toe but does not relieve the metatarsus primus varus (Fig. 8–25).[31, 32]

Arthrodesis of the first metatarsophalangeal joint, performed to relieve the valgus

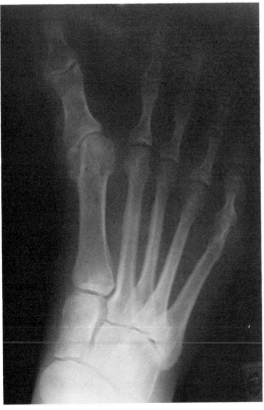

**Figure 8–21.** Congenital hallux varus is characterized by medial angulation of the great toe at the metatarsophalangeal joint.

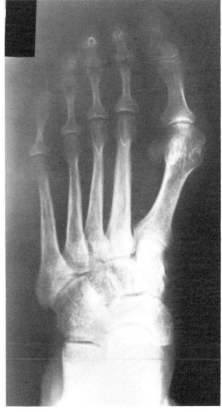

**Figure 8–22.** Hallux valgus is characterized by medial angulation of the first metatarsal, lateral angulation of the proximal phalanx, and lateral displacement of the sesamoids.

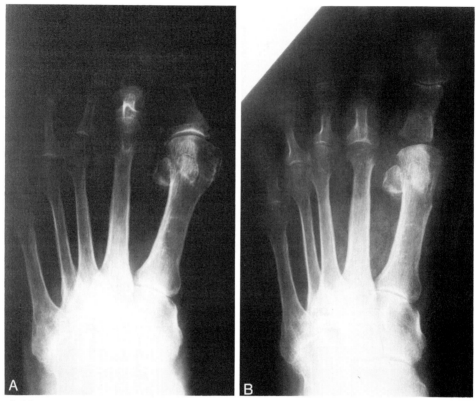

**Figure 8–23.** *A,* Hallux valgus bunion deformity and hammer toe deformities, 2nd, 3rd and 4th toes. *B,* Keller bunionectomy and hemiphalangectomy, 2nd, 3rd, and 5th toes. (Courtesy of Dr. Gilbert Shapiro, Tucson, Arizona.)

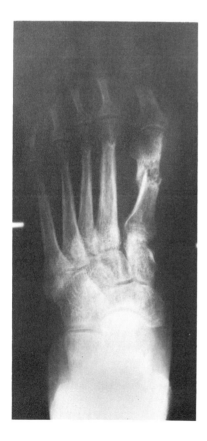

**Figure 8–24.** A metatarsal osteotomy has been performed to correct the varus deformity (same patient as in Figure 8–22).

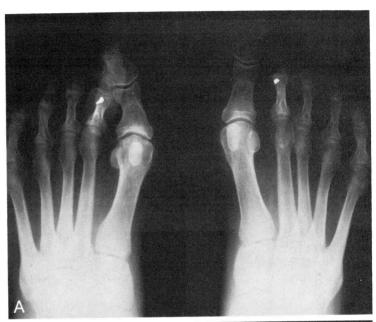

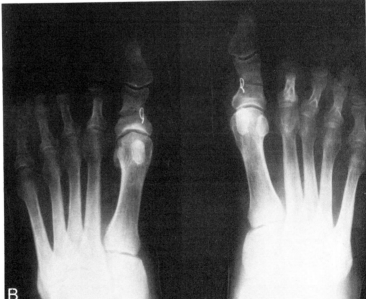

**Figure 8–25.** Bilateral osteotomies have been performed to correct valgus deformity of the great toe as well as hemiphalangectomies of the second toe for hammer toe deformity. (Courtesy of Dr. Gilbert Shapiro, Tucson, Arizona.)

deformity, may also be utilized when other operative procedures fail.[33, 34]

## Dorsal Bunion

This deformity is thought to be due to muscle imbalance resulting in a spur that forms on the dorsal aspect of the first metatarsal head and to an associated bursitis. The deformity consists of dorsiflexion of the first metatarsophalangeal joint and plantar flexion of the interphalangeal joint. Treatment is surgical, consisting of tendon transfer or arthrodesis if the deformity is severe. Arthrodesis may include the first metatarso-cuneiform, navicular-cuneiform, and the first metatarsophalangeal joint.

## Flatfoot

A flatfoot deformity is characterized by a decrease in or loss of the normal longitudinal arch that develops after birth.[24, 35]

The longitudinal arch, most prominent in the medial aspect of the foot, is dependent upon the talocalcaneal axial relationship as well as adequate muscle tone and ligamentous support.

Flatfoot may be of the hypermobile type, related to ligamentous or muscle laxity, in which the arch is restored on non–weight-bearing, or of the rigid type, related to bony, cartilaginous, or fibrous bridges between the talus and the calcaneus or between the talus and the navicular (Fig. 8–26).[36–38]

In the lateral projection the increased talocalcaneal angle is seen in which the longi-

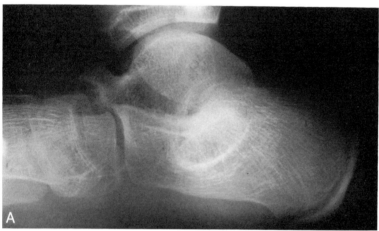

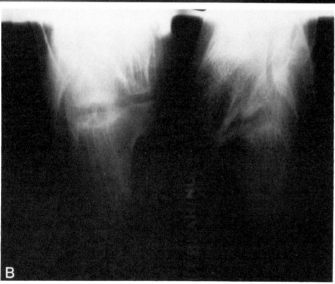

**Figure 8–26.** Flatfoot. *A,* Weight-bearing lateral view demonstrates loss of the normal longitudinal arch in a patient with a rigid flat foot. Calcaneal beaking indicates tarsal coalition as the cause. *B,* Axial views indicate incomplete talocalcaneal fusion on the left.

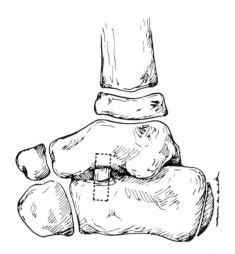

**Figure 8–27.** Grice procedure is characterized by bony struts lateral to and bridging the talocalcaneal joint.

tudinal axis through the talus is directed inferiorly to the base of the first metatarsal. An increased talocalcaneal angle in the anteroposterior projection shows that the longitudinal axis through the talus runs medial to the first metatarsal.[20]

Surgical treatment, utilized when the disability is severe, includes an extra-articular arthrodesis or triple arthrodesis. The extra-articular arthrodesis (Grice procedure) utilizes bony struts lateral to the talocalcaneal joint and therefore not interfering with growth of the foot. Fusion usually occurs within six weeks (Fig. 8–27).[39, 40] A triple arthrodesis is utilized once full growth has been achieved (Fig. 8–28).

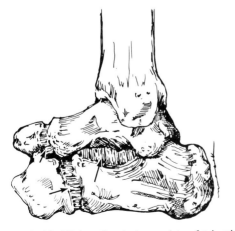

**Figure 8–28.** Triple arthrodesis consists of talocalcaneal, talonavicular and calcaneocuboid fusion (arrows).

## Cavus Foot (Pes Cavus)

Cavus foot or pes cavus deformity commonly results from paralytic and central nervous system disorders (polio, Charcot-Marie-Tooth, Friedreich's ataxia) owing to muscle paralysis and imbalance. It is characterized by an accentuated high longitudinal arch and an equinus position of the forefoot. Tendon transfers are effective in correcting deformities before the foot attains full growth. Once full growth has been attained, however, bony procedures are necessary to maintain alignment and stabilization.

In the lateral projection there is an increased talocalcaneal angle (Fig. 8–29). The longitudinal axis through the talus is directed superiorly to the first metatarsal. The anteroposterior projection shows a decreased talocalcaneal angle.

The treatment of pes cavus is surgical if the deformity is progressive. Soft tissue releases are performed in children to avoid interference with growth of the foot and before fixed bony structural changes have resulted. Once fixed bone deformity has resulted, surgery on the underlying bone is necessary.

A posterior calcaneal osteotomy (Dwyer procedure) may be performed to shift the heel from varus into valgus. This procedure may be utilized during the active growth period.[41]

A V-osteotomy (tarsal osteotomy of Japas) may be performed to correct the equinus deformity of the foot. The apex of the osteotomy is at the highest point of the cavus deformity, usually in the navicular, and extends distally through the cuboid and first cuneiform.[42]

An anterior tarsal wedge osteotomy may be performed in the adult foot, but not the actively growing foot, because shortening of the foot results. It spares, therefore allowing mobility of, the talonavicular and calcaneocuboid joints. A wedge osteotomy is performed with the apex in the cuboid and extends through the navicular in its proximal aspect and through the tarsal bones in its distal aspect, depending on the thickness of the wedge required to correct the equinus deformity.[43]

During the early stage of the deformity, fusion of the first metatarsocuneiform or first

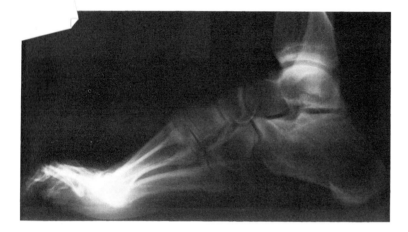

**Figure 8–29.** Pes cavus deformity is recognized by accentuation of the longitudinal arch and equinus position of the forefoot. This is a patient with Charcot-Marie-Tooth disease (peroneal muscle atrophy).

metatarsocuneiform-navicular joints may be performed to correct the cavus deformity.[44]

A severe pes cavus deformity may require a combination of surgical procedures to correct the fixed structural changes that have occurred. These include a wedge osteotomy, triple arthrodesis, Jones procedure of the great toe (extensor tendon transfer to first metatarsal, straightening and fusion of the interphalangeal joint) and resection of the metatarsal heads, and straightening and fusion of the proximal interphalangeal joints of the other toes.

### Tarsal Coalition

Tarsal coalition was previously mentioned as a cause of rigid flatfoot. Those cases not responding to conservative treatment may require surgical intervention. If a talocalcaneal bar is present, a talocalcaneal fusion is performed. If the coalition is fibrous or cartilaginous, rendering the subtalar joint unstable, a subtalar fusion is performed in addition to a talonavicular fusion.

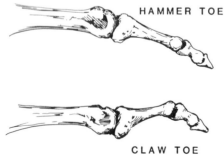

HAMMER TOE

CLAW TOE

**Figure 8–30.** Diagram of hammer and claw toes.

### Hammer Toe and Claw Toe

A hammer toe is characterized by flexion at the proximal interphalangeal joint, in contrast to claw toe, which consists of flexion at the proximal interphalangeal joint and hyperextension of the metatarsophalangeal joint (Fig. 8–30).

The purpose of treatment, which is surgical, is to correct the deformity, allowing the patient to wear stylish shoes and to eliminate pressure points for callus formation.

Radiographic appearance of the surgical correction of the hammer toe is characterized by excision of the base of the distal phalanx and head of the proximal phalanx, maintenance of alignment by intramedullary pin fixation, and subsequent fusion (see Fig. 8–23B).

Surgical correction of clawing of the great toe is characterized by wedge resection and arthrodesis of the proximal interphalangeal joint (Jones procedure). Correction of the deformity in the other toes consists of resection of the base of the proximal phalanx and the interphalangeal joints and maintenance of alignment with intramedullary pins.[45]

### Hallux Rigidus

This condition is characterized by painful restricted motion of the first metatarsophalangeal joint.

The radiographic appearance is that of degenerative arthritis, but the radiograph may be normal or may demonstrate a large

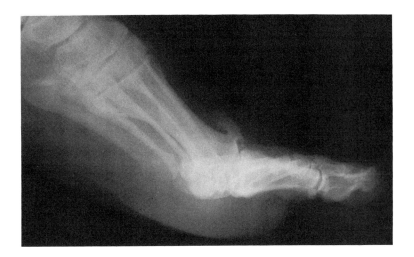

**Figure 8–31.** Hallux rigidus.

exostosis on the dorsum of the head of the first metatarsal (Fig. 8–31).

The treatment of hallux rigidus is variable, therefore influencing the postoperative radiograph. Keller arthroplasty involves resection of a considerable portion of the base of the proximal phalanx. Arthrodesis consists of metatarsophalangeal joint fusion. Osteotomy and depression of the first metatarsal segment may be performed in association with an arthroplasty. Flexible implant arthroplasty replaces the base of the proximal phalanx with a flexible silicone rubber implant (Fig. 8–32).[46]

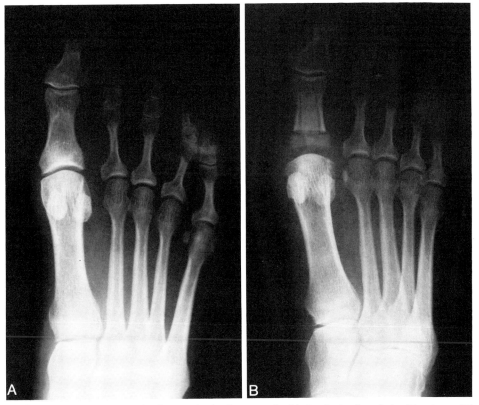

**Figure 8–32.** *A* and *B*, Treatment of hallux rigidus by Swanson flexible implant arthroplasty. (Courtesy of Dr. Gilbert Shapiro, Tucson, Arizona.)

**es**

1. Leonard MH: Injuries of the lateral ligaments of the ankle—a clinical and experimental study. J Bone Joint Surg 31A:373–377, 1949
2. Turek SL: The foot and ankle. *In* Turek SL: Orthopaedics: Principles and their Application. 3rd ed. J.B. Lippincott Co., Philadelphia, 1977, pp. 1245–1321
3. Olson RW: Arthrography of the ankle: its use in the evaluation of ankle sprains. Radiology 92:1439–1446, 1969
4. Brostrom L, Liljeahl SO, Lindvall N: II. Arthrographic diagnosis of recent ligament ruptures. Acta Chir Scand 129:485–499, 1965
5. Ruth CJ: The surgical treatment of injuries of the fibular collateral ligaments of the ankle. J Bone Joint Surg 43A:229–239, 1961
6. Gaston S, McLaughlin HL: Complex fracture of the lateral malleolus. J Trauma 1:69–78, 1961
7. Cave EF: Fracture of the os calcis: the problem in general. Clin Orthop 30:64–66, 1963
8. Giannestras NJ, Samniarco GJ: Fractures and dislocations in the foot. *In* Rockwood CA, Green DP: Fractures. J.B. Lippincott, Philadelphia, 1975, pp. 1400–1495
9. Resnick D, Georgen TG: Peroneal tenography in previous calcaneal fractures. Radiology 115:211–213, 1975
10. Deyerle WM: Long term follow-up of fractures of the os calcis. Diagnostic peroneal synoviagram. Orthop Clin N Am 4:213–227, 1973
11. Newberg AH: Osteochondral fractures of the dome of the talus. Br J Radiol 52:105–109, 1979
12. McKaever FM: Fracture of the neck of the astragalus. Arch Surg 46:720–735, 1943
13. McKaever FM: Treatment and complications of fractures and dislocations of the talus. Clin Orthop 30:45–52, 1963
14. Pennal GF: Fractures of the talus. Clin Orthop 30:53–63, 1963
15. Garcia A, Parkes JC: II: Fractures of the foot. *In* Giannestras NJ: Foot Disorders, Medical and Surgical Management. 2nd ed. Lea and Febiger, Philadelphia, 1973
16. Burwell HN, Charnley AD: The treatment of displaced fractures at the ankle by rigid internal fixation and early joint movement. J Bone Joint Surg 47B:634–660, 1965
17. Klossner O: Late results of operative and non-operative treatment of severe ankle fractures. Acta Chir Scand (Suppl.) 293:1–93, 1962 [Vasli S: Operative treatment of ankle fractures. Acta Chir Scand (Suppl.) 226:1–74, 1957]
18. Wilson FC, Skilbred LA: Long-term results in treatment of displaced bimalleolar fractures. J Bone Joint Surg 48A:1065–1073, 1966
19. Buchholtz, HW: Complications of arthroplasty and total joint replacement in the ankle. *In* Epps CH (ed): Complication in Orthopedic Surgery. Vol. 2. J.B. Lippincott Co., Philadelphia, 1978, pp. 979–994
20. Condon VR: Radiology of practical orthopedic problems. Radiol Clin N Am 10:203–223, 1972
21. Keim HA, Ritchie GW: Weight-bearing roentgenograms in the evaluation of foot deformities. Clin Orthop 70:133–136, 1970
22. Swann M, Lloyd-Roberts GC, Catterall A: The anatomy of uncorrected club feet. J Bone Joint Surg 51B:263–269, 1969
23. Coleman SS, Stelling FH, III, Jarrett J: Pathomechanics and treatment of congenital vertical talus. Clin Orthop 70:62–72, 1970
24. Ginannestras NJ: Recognition and treatment of flatfeet in infancy. Clin Orthop 70:10–29, 1970
25. Danes-Colley N: Contraction of the metatarsophalangeal joint of the great toe. Br Med J 1:728, 1887
26. Bingham R: The Stone operation for hallux valgus. Chir Orthop 17:366, 1960
27. Mayo CH: The surgical treatment of bunions. Ann Surg 48:300, 1908
28. Keller WL: Surgical treatment of bunions and hallux valgus. NY Med J 80:741, 1904
29. Lapidus PW: Operative correction of the metatarsus varus primus in hallux valgus. Surg Gynecol Obstet 58:183, 1934
30. Mitchell CL, et al: Osteotomy-bunionectomy for hallux valgus. J Bone Joint Surg 40A:41, 1958
31. Butterworth RD, Clary BB: A bunion operation. VA Med Montly 90:11, 1963
32. Colloff B, Weitz EM: Proximal phalangeal osteotomy in hallux valgus. Clin Orthop 54:105, 1967
33. McKeever DC: Arthrodesis of the first metatarsophalangeal joint for hallux valgus, hallux rigidus, and metatarsus primus varus. J Bone Joint Surg 34A:129, 1952
34. Thompson FR, McElvenny RT: Arthrodesis of the first metatarsophalangeal joint. J Bone Joint Surg 22:55, 1940
35. Ritchie GW, Keim HA: Major foot deformities—their classification and x-ray analysis. J Canad Assoc Radiol 19:155–166, 1969
36. LeLievre J: Current concepts and correction in the valgus foot. Clin Orthop 70:43–53, 1970
37. Mitchell GP: Spasmodic flatfoot. Clin Orthop 70:75–78, 1970
38. Harris RI: Retrospect-peroneal spastic flatfoot (rigid valgus foot). J Bone Joint Surg 47A:1657–1667, 1965
39. Grice DS: An extra-articular arthrodesis of the subastragalar joint for correction of paralytic flatfeet in children. J Bone Joint Surg 34A:927, 1952
40. Grice DS: Further experience with extra-articular arthrodesis of the subtalar joint. J Bone Joint Surg 37A:246, 1955
41. Dwyer FC: Osteotomy of calcaneum for pes cavus. J Bone Joint Surg 41B:80, 1959
42. Japas LM: Surgical treatment of pes cavus by tarsal V-osteotomy. J Bone Joint Surg 50A:927, 1968
43. Cole WH: The treatment of clawfoot. J Bone Joint Surg 22:895, 1940
44. McElvenny RT, Caldwell GD: A new operation for correction of cavus foot. Clin Orthop 11:85, 1958
45. Jones R: The soldier's foot and the treatment of common deformities of the foot. II. Claw-foot. Br Med J 1:749, 1961
46. Swanson AB: Implant arthroplasty for the great toe. Clin Orthop 85:75, 1972

# INDEX

Note: Page numbers in italics refer to illustrations; those followed by the letter "t" indicate tables.

**BUSINESS REPLY CARD**

FIRST CLASS   PERMIT NO. 101   PHILADELPHIA, PA

POSTAGE WILL BE PAID BY ADDRESSEE

# W.B. SAUNDERS COMPANY

west washington square
philadelphia, pa 19105-9967

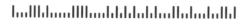